*Plan your rehab,
and follow your plan . . .
to Success!*

Effective Orthopedic Rehab

Seven Steps to Complete Recovery

Buck Willis, Ph.D., ACSM

Printed in Victoria, Canada

National Library of Canada Cataloguing in Publication Data

Willis, Buck, 1964-
    Effective orthopedic rehab : seven steps to complete recovery / Buck Willis.
ISBN 1-4120-0522-1
    I. Title.
RD797.W44 2003   616.7'03   C2003-903349-X

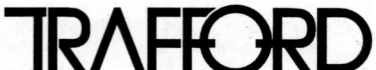

This book was published *on-demand* in cooperation with Trafford Publishing.
On-demand publishing is a unique process and service of making a book available for retail sale to the public taking advantage of on-demand manufacturing and Internet marketing.
On-demand publishing includes promotions, retail sales, manufacturing, order fulfilment, accounting and collecting royalties on behalf of the author.

Suite 6E, 2333 Government St., Victoria, B.C. V8T 4P4, CANADA
Phone   250-383-6864   Toll-free   1-888-232-4444 (Canada & US)
Fax   250-383-6804   E-mail   sales@trafford.com
Web site   www.trafford.com   TRAFFORD PUBLISHING IS A DIVISION OF TRAFFORD HOLDINGS LTD.
Trafford Catalogue #03-0891   www.trafford.com/robots/03-0891.html

10   9   8   7   6   5   4   3   2

Acknowledgements

In writing this book I am continually thankful for the loving, caring family members and health care providers that helped me find such success following my traumatic plane crash. Thanks to Mom, Dad, Deborah, Dr. Spears, Dr. Reynolds, Dr. Turner, Dr. Smith, Dr. Bagwell, Dr. Bissett, and all of the other great people who helped me to stand, walk and eventually find greater emotional strength than I had ever had before the crash!

Then I wish to sincerely thank my teachers and academic colleagues who helped me pursue growth, academically and emotionally through my learning of kinesiology, athletic training, and medicine. Let me offer my sincere thanks to Dr. Burkhardt, Dr. Walker, Dr. Johnson, Dr. Glassman, Dr. Gravitt, and Patch Adams, MD.

My dear wife Adele has stood by me through many challenges, and she even helped my complete rehabilitation by being the best-friend + true-partner + confidant + true-love that I had always dreamt of finding! Thank you Nani, *MTL FAAD!*

My greatest thanks goes to the greatest healer and greatest teacher of all times;

Thank you God!

Effective Orthopedic Rehab
Seven Steps to Complete Recovery

TABLE OF CONTENTS

Introduction

This book will reveal the seven key steps to obtaining complete orthopedic rehabilitation. These steps are effective for any orthopedic anomaly from a sprained ankle to rehabilitation from multiple, complex fractures and surgeries, which the author experienced after suffering an "Unsurvivable, traumatic plane crash."

The introduction will describe the full picture of rehabilitation from designing one's rehabilitation program to proactive exercises for preventing injury reoccurrence. Then this chapter will reveal success that people have gained from following Dr. Willis' seven rehab steps.

The seven steps to complete rehabilitation are as follows:
I   Injury Analysis
II Setting Rehab Goals
III Determine the Components for Rehab Success
IV Examine the Current Exercise Therapies
V   Design and Follow your own Rehabilitation Program
VI Measure Progress to Determine Completion of Goals and Rehab
VII Proactive Exercises and Lifestyle Fitness

Components of Rehab Design

Components for rehabilitation design begin with prioritizing goals for immediate treatment, which include the following:
1) Decreasing the symptoms,
2) Regaining complete range of motion (ROM),
3) Neuromuscular Control,
4) Flexibility training, and
5) Strength training.

1

One must immediately treat the injury with techniques to reduce the pain, inflammation, and swelling if present after the injury.

Rehabilitation must be done in different *phases* to ensure safety and a logical progression in the rehabilitation so that the recovery is permanent and complete. A frequent question asked is "When does one start the rehabilitation after an injury" and "How fast should rehab progress?" The answers to these questions are "Immediately" and "For rehab, use the cadence of *Safety First*."

For instance, after surgical repair of a torn Anterior Cruciate (knee) Ligament, the post-operative treatment begins by placing the patient's leg into a kinetic, motion device, (so the knee is continually being gently flexed and extended), even before the patient regains consciousness. This book will show how to reduce the symptoms of an orthopedic injury and begin rehab with conservative motion protocols in the appropriate *phases* of rehabilitation.

Phases in Rehabilitation

The Phases are the appropriate therapeutic exercises with proper timing for the best recuperation. In Chapter IV, the book will address common injuries/conditions, (with lists of the symptoms), and then it will thoroughly describe the Rehab *Phases* that are appropriate in treating each injury.

Acute phase is the treatment suggested for the first 1 to 3 days where the primary goals are focused on the reduction of pain, inflammation, and swelling. Techniques like Rest, Ice, Compression, and Elevation (*RICE*), will be used, and in this phase, one may only begin with gentle work on ROM. For example, in the case of treating *Pitcher's elbow*, the elbow would be wrapped with an elastic bandage, ice packs would be applied, and the elbow would be elevated above the heart's level. Then in specific training sessions, one would only gently flex the elbow through pain-free angles of motion, and utilize passive, static stretching.

The *Rehab phase* normally occurs from day 4 to approximately day 14 after the injury occurred. In this phase, one works to regain complete ROM and neuromuscular control, while beginning light, progressive resistance, with continued flexibility training. In the case of an elbow injury, the *Rehab phase* would include stretching of the wrist, elbow, and shoulder muscles, and will begin regaining neuromuscular control, (which is select muscle activation and sensation from that muscle's contraction). In this *Phase,* unique beneficial exercises like controlled elbow extension exercises can be performed, and the exercise would be fully described with pictures. (See page 64-67.) One would also begin isometric contractions which are muscle contractions without moving the limb.

One's *Recovery phase* works for regaining full function of the injured area, and focuses on progressive resistance, which allows one to also pursue treating the cause of the injury. Flexibility training will be continued, this phase can continue for several more weeks. For the "Tennis elbow" injury, the *Recovery phase* will address strengthening the weaker muscles, such as brachioradialis, because an imbalance in the elbow musculature may have caused this disorder, [6] (see figure #4, pg 62). Training for muscular balance will be accomplished using unique exercises to include weight balancing, and hammer rotation for the *Recovery phase* for tennis elbow.

Then after each phase's exercises have been explained and illustrated with pictures, each section will close with a possible outline of treatment, such as this:

Tennis Elbow Rehab summary
Acute phase: FIRST 3 DAYS
(RICE) Rest, Ice,
Compression,
Elevation
Passive, Static Stretching
Rehab phase: DAY 4 to 2nd WEEK
Isometric contractions
Elbow Extension across chest
Recovery: WEEKS 3 to 6
Hammer rotation
Joystick rotation
Overhead Medicine Ball

3

Complete Rehabilitation

Complete rehabilitation must include the prioritized goals listed below, and while the list may seem vast, these priorities are easily accomplished in harmony with the proper, consecutive Rehab Phases.

1. Reduced pain, inflammation, and swelling
2. Healing of the tissue
3. Regain the joint's range of motion (ROM)
4. Increased blood flow
5. Restore complete neuromuscular control of the injured area
6. Counteract tendencies for muscle atrophy
7. Regain and increase strength and power
8. Reactivate and ensure the proprioceptive abilities, (sensation of muscle contraction), and
9. Regain and increase endurance for sport and normal activities

However, if these priorities for rehabilitation are not accomplished, the injured person may suffer from muscle atrophy (loss of muscle size and strength), and the decrease in muscle fibers' diameter, which will result in weakness, and decreased muscular endurance. If one chooses to treat an orthopedic injury with inactivity, it could yield significant muscle atrophy, such as a 40% decrease muscle mass in just three weeks. [1]

Twenty five exercise therapies prescribed for known, common orthopedic injuries will be described, and these therapies include 72 stretching protocols and 112 strength training protocols. If you have an injury other than what is listed, then you will be given the tools to design your own program. The list or protocols are also there for you to use when modifying the exercises in your final phase of *Recovery* rehabilitation.

Rehabilitation Success from Dr. Willis' *Rehab Steps*

The following stories show the tremendous success from using the author's Effective Orthopedic Rehab Steps. The Author's initial experience was designing and implementing a rehab program for himself, following what the FAA called an "Unsurvivable, traumatic plane crash" and the resulting 16 operations that lasted over three years. (See cover photo.) This included rehabilitation following each of the 16 operation on his legs, and a three-month duration of open wound, chloral-hydrotherapy to clean the tarsal bones of a frequently fatal bone infection, *osteomyelitis.*

The author's rehab efforts paid off. After the tremendous care from his team of physicians and surgeons, he achieved success in competitive mountain-bike racing and success in graduate school with research on the biomechanical components of orthopedic rehabilitation. His goal is to use his knowledge and experience to help and serve others.

Another powerful success story from using the author's rehabilitation steps belongs to a woman who had a traumatic head injury with comminuted fractures of her lower legs, when she was 36. This woman took the rehab challenge with enthusiasm, and her success following the Author's Seven Steps has included placing in a Fitness competition, and completing her education to become a Registered Nurse. She now cares for older patients who have had brain damage from strokes (cerebral infarctions), and her background gives her the tools of empathy and rehab success.

She also used the techniques described in this book to help her through another difficult and exhausting experience of regaining her fitness after pregnancy. She successfully regained her abdominal lines in just four months after delivering (post-partum), and she credits the conditioning steps that she learned from the author, because it "fueled" her interest in continued exercise and now she is a successful, competitive tri-athlete.

A few years ago, a woman who was in college to become a commercial pilot had a traumatic car accident. She had a severely injured ankle that required a total fusion of her medial anklebones for permanent immobilization (*tarsal arthrodesis*),

5

just as the author required after his plane crash. She had abandoned her goals of becoming a commercial pilot, until she read of the author's success in the March 2001 issue of *AOPA Pilot*. She then contacted the author and followed his advice and "Steps" for complete rehabilitation through her operations and following physical therapy. This woman is now a commercial Pilot, and a Flight Instructor Pilot!

How will you design the Rehab for your own strong success?

To answer this challenging question, follow the key seven steps and ask yourself these questions:

I. Injury analysis: How severe is your injury, and where are you hurt the worst?

II. Setting your rehab goals: What do you want to accomplish and in what order?

III. Determine the components to be used in your rehab: Is regaining flexibility or strength your top priority?

IV. Examine the current therapeutic exercises: What protocols would be most beneficial and relevant to your injury and your goals?

V. Design and follow your rehab plan: Have you left room for changes in your plan, and are you prepared for the rehab plateaus or set-backs that will occur?

VI. Measure progress and completion of your rehab & goals: When have you reached the small and large goals, and when should you reset your goals?

VII. Proactive exercise and lifestyle fitness: What exercises will help deter reoccurrence?

One will find the answers to these rehab questions in the following seven chapters.

Chapter I
Injury Analysis

===

Severity and *R.I.C.E.*

The first step for the individual and/or health care provider is to immediately treat the injury so that it does not worsen and then one should analyze the **severity** of the injury. The initial treatment that reduces symptoms and keeps the injury form progressing is to use *RICE*, and that acronym stands for "Rest," "Ice," "Compression," and "Elevation." The faster that these techniques can be administered to an orthopedic injury, the less likely the injury is to progress, and this will help reduce inflammation, swelling, and pain.

Applying an ice pack or a bag of frozen peas to the injured area can be done over an elastic, compression bandage. Ace® bandage works well but, make sure that it is not too tight because stopping the blood flow completely will cause tissue death (necrosis). Then tape or secure an ice pack to the injured, inflamed area, and elevate the injured area in any way possible. (For a picture showing an ankle wrap see picture #43, page 102.)

If it was not a traumatic or acute injury, the individual may also have to decide when it would be appropriate to consult their physicians, physical therapists, etc., and the following information will help you to make an informed decision. The key factors to determine the severity of the injury will be:

1) Inflammation, Swelling, (Edema)
2) Mobility changes and restrictions (motor performance change and weight bearing or load-carrying abilities
3) Pain, and
4) Visual examination and Imagery

If the injury was not severe enough to warrant a hospital visit then people often question if their injury or chronic pain is severe enough to warrant consultation with a physician. To find that answer, use the following questions:

- Is the swelling consistent or does it go down after using *RICE* for 30 minutes?
- Is there bruising and how much of the area is darkly discolored?
- Are you able to move the injured joint at all?

- If you can move your joint, is the movement less than half of your normal range of motion?
- If it is a leg, ankle or foot injury, can you stand on both feet with your weight distributed evenly?
- If you can stand on both feet, can you lift your uninjured foot/leg just for an instant?
- Does the pain throb or does is it a sharp, cutting pain?

- Will the swelling go down overnight?

If you answered affirmatively to many of these questions, then you should definitely see a physician, so that they can diagnosis and/or rule out fractures and torn ligaments or tendons, etc. That is because those conditions that were not examined by a physician and go untreated, may cause lifetime disabilities. If you are not in the category where you need to seek immediate medical care, you should still keep a log of your pain and symptoms so that you can communicate it effectively to a health care provider, should you decide later to seek their help.

The most common and most frequent injuries that happen in athletics are the Sprain, Strain, and Contusion injuries. [2,7,10,14,15] A sprain is an injurious stretch or tear in a ligament (connects bone to bone), where as a strain is a similar injury to one's tendon that connects bone to muscle. A contusion injury is normally an impact injury where later there is bleeding in the tissue beneath the skin causing bruising. A clinical example of the difference would be comparing an ankle sprain vs. a knee contusion vs. tennis elbow.

When one twists an ankle or has a lateral ankle sprain (see picture on page 101), the ligaments that connect the anklebones, (the carpal bones such as the calcaneus) are excessively stretched or torn. If one is playing football or soccer and one receives a severe side-blow to the knee, it would be called a contusion injury, and bruising (bleeding beneath the skin) can be expected. However, if the blow was extreme enough or if the blow caused you to then hyperextend the knee, a Cruciate Ligament tear could be the result. The ankle and knee injuries described are ligament injuries.

Tennis elbow is an example of chronic tendon inflammation and another injury on that tendon could cause it to tear or rupture. The tendon is the elastic tissue that connects muscle to bone, (such as the extensor muscles of the lower arm with the epicondyl of the humerus). Lower back injuries are also commonly tendon strains or tears because the injury occurs where the deep back muscles such as spinal erector muscles attach to the vertebra.

The intensity of pain and characteristic symptoms often reveal how acute or severe the injury was. For example:

- A Mild Ankle Sprain would not have bruising or ankle instability.
- Moderate Ankle Sprain the athlete would hear a "Pop" as he "rolled over" or twisted the injured ankle. The pain would be more severe and point-specific, and bruising would occur in a day or two.
- A Severe Ankle Sprain would also have a "Pop" sound followed by ankle instability, (Ankle instability is when the ankle bones would subluxate or slide in and out of place) and the pain would be both point-specific and over the entire ankle area. It would be difficult or impossible to walk or even stand on this severely sprained ankle.

Analysis of the Pain

One's pain is the most obvious component that we are trying to reduce, alleviate, and prevent from occurring again. A joint injury will make the area around the joint red, inflamed, painful, and will yield a change in movement or flexibility from the inflammation and swelling (edema). There are several *Pain Scales* that often ask the sufferer to rate their pain from a range of zero to eleven. This helps the person suffering the pain to discriminate, which helps them evaluate their recovery and progression from the acute stages of an injury. However, the best and most complete instrument for analyzing pain comes from the book, *Chronic Pain Evaluation: a valid, standardized assessment instrument,* by Dr. Karen S. Rucker. Dr. Rucker's assessment is very effective, analytical instrument for measuring pain, and it has been verified with several studies.

The author has changed that form, into a 110-point pain scale for your needs of pain assessment. You can copy this form or write down your answers on a separate piece of paper, so that you can use this test later for progression and to measure the change in your pain as your rehabilitation continues. This form will give you the *Pre* and *Post* feedback to help gauge one's progress towards complete rehabilitation.

Pain Assessment Test

Date _____
Date of injury or onset of pain _____

1. Is pain your primary health problem? ___
       Yes (2 points), No (0 points)

2. Does the pain radiate to other areas? ___
       Yes = 1, No = 0

3. Is the pain in a small point or a large area? ___
       Point = 1, Area = 2

4. Is the pain on the surface or deep? ___
       Deep = 2, Surface = 1

Pain Frequency

5. In the past 6 weeks how often have you had pain?
    0 = Every other week   1 = Once a week   2 = Once a day
    3 = many times each day

6. How often since your injury or onset of pain, have you been pain free?
       3 = minutes, 2 = hours, 1 = days, 0 = weeks

7. How long does the pain last?
       4 = more than a day continuously, 3 = for hours continuously, 2 = only an hour,
       1 = less than an hour, 0 = only when I over exert

10

8. In the past 6 weeks what time of day is your pain the worst? (Note this specifically for diagnosis of different problems).

> 1 = always the same, 2 = When you first get up, 3 = Only afternoon, 4 = Both day & night

9. In the past 6 weeks does the pain make it hard to get to sleep?

> 0 = Never, 1 = Some nights, 2 = most nights

10. In the past 6 weeks, how often does your pain awaken you?

> 0 = Never, 1 = After you have participated in sports that day, 2 = Frequently

11. How difficult is it to cope with your pain?

> 0 = Easy to deal with, 1 = Inconvenient, 2 = troublesome, 3 = Almost impossible

12. How much does the pain interfere with your athletics or with weight-bearing activities?

> 1 = Only occasionally, 2 = frequently, 3 = Every time you have excessive movement
> 4 = Anytime that you are active

14. How often do you take medication for your pain?

> 0 = Less than once a week, 1 = Several times per week, 2 = Once Daily, 3 = More than once every day, since the injury

PAIN SEVERITY

13. Please check the columns below that describe how much your pain affects you in different conditions.

Activity	0 = none	1 = little	3 = Moderate	4 = Severe
Standing				
Walking				
Sitting				
Lifting weights				
Pulling/Pushing				
Climbing stairs				
Descending stairs				
Stooping				
Kneeling				
Rotation				
Swinging				
Running				
Throwing				
Twisting torso				
Reaching up				
Squatting (0 lbs)				

15. Describe the medications' affect on your pain.
   0 = It always stops the pain, 1 = Decreases the pain, 2 = Usually takes the pain
   away, 4 = Little or no affect on the pain

16. How does the pain affect you emotionally?
   0 = No affect, 1 = It causes anxiety, 2 = The pain worries me daily, 4 = It makes me
   consider giving up my recreational activities

17. Rate the limitations that your pain/injury affects your daily life style.

> 0 = Does not limit your lifestyle,
> 1 = some activities avoided (i.e. riding in car or sitting in stadium for hours),
> 3 = You avoid all activity due to injury

18. Now calculate and record your total score of pain assessment. _____

List the unique times that pain occurs:

_____

_____

_____

_____

If you feel that your answers are high in this scale, then you should take your test results to a qualified physician who can give you information and/or treatment about your injury and pain. Use the following nurse's acronym, *OLD CHART* to track your progression and, one can also use this to determine the pain intensity and also help to determine the injury's severity. [13]

Onset (when did it begin and what were you doing)
Location (home, work, or athletics)
Duration *(how long at the first onset, and how long are you in pain now)*
Characteristics of pain ("sharp, shooting" pain vs. "dull throbbing")
Aggravating factors (such as certain movement triggers the pain or pain with compression)
Radiation (what areas are feeling the pain) Further radiation means greater severity of injury
Treatment (what is effective or ineffective in treating the pain)

Inflammation, Swelling

Inflammation is a localized response to injury or damage to tissue, and it is a control mechanism to immediately send assistance to the injured tissue. Inflammation has increased blood flow with dilated arterioles and capillaries, which often results in the warm, reddening of the inflamed area. Unfortunately, increased blood flow to an extremity is often accompanied by swelling (edema).

Edema is the restriction of venous blood flow and such "swelling" is the body's control method of decreasing the spread of an injury and, it may also be the natural accumulation of fluid used to treat the injury. RICE, (previously described), effectively treats swelling and inflammation. An example of these symptoms would be after one acutely twisted or "sprained" one's ankle. The person might have felt or heard a "pop" and then the ankle was painful to walk on and may have required assistance for ambulation or movement. The ankle may be causing acute, or high levels of pain, and that could be assisted by anti-inflammatory medications like ibuprofen or Celebrex®.

Mobility Restrictions

If there is a change in mobility it may be due to an injury where the muscle and tendons have been injured or damaged severely, but it may also be an injury of ligaments and or bone tissue. In either case the mobility change is very useful in identifying the severity of the injury.

When an injury has occurred, one can test the muscle and tendons by using isometric contractions. This means that you will flex the muscle in a manner where you do not move the limb, and your opposing muscles are providing the resistance against movement. For example, when one flexes the quadriceps muscles while concurrently flexing the hamstring muscles, the muscles tighten but the limb does not move. Another example would be to put one's hands beneath a heavy desk, and flex the biceps muscles, but use the weight of the table to inhibit the movement.

14

PASSIVE MOVEMENT TEST is one where the limb moves without the muscle contraction, and this tests for injury to ligament or bony tissue. For example, if you can relax and let a partner lift your arm, it would be passive movement. Can this be done without pain? If a partner raises your hand and then you simply let it fall with gravity as the activating force, this would PASSIVELY test to see if there was a ligament or bone injury in the upper arm or shoulder.

Visual Examination

One key component to a physical examination is the physical appearance of the injured area, and this is used as a diagnostic tool in many cases. If the area is bruised or obtusely swollen a health professional might immediately suspect a fracture or torn connective tissue and send the patient for X-ray or Magnetic Resonance Imaging (MRI). If an unusual appearance is part of your injury, you must immediately seek medical care.

Chapter II
Setting the Rehab Goals

The first step was to determine the severity of your injury and the second step is to begin setting rehab goals. However, to set your goals of rehab progression, you have to know your starting point, and this will help give you feedback as you evaluate your progress through the 7 rehab steps described on page 1. So begin by testing your Range of motion (extension, flexion, and rotation), your strength, and your endurance.

Initial tests

• Range of Motion
Measure the degree of extension, flexion, and rotation that is possible before you start treating your injury. For example, if you have a knee disorder, determine if you can fully extend your knee to the "locked" position of 180°. Then measure your flexibility to see how much you can contract or "close" the joint angle. For example when your leg is totally extended it is 180° and normal knee flexion is to an angle of 30 to 40 degrees. To measure this (i.e. knee injury), lie on your back with your leg extended up into the air. Now, flex the knee and measure the distance from your heel to your buttocks. For an elbow injury perform the same flexibility test measuring from wrist to shoulder.

Note the distance between your heel and middle thigh or from your heel to your buttocks (gluteus muscles). Obviously the different lengths of each person's limbs will make this measurement different, but you are testing your own flexibility.

Then also measure the rotation that you can do obtain, and to do this imagine that your foot in the normal, anatomical position to be pointing towards 12 o'clock on a watch. Then measure and record the position with your toes pointing furthest to the right and furthest to the left, based on clock numbering. Then measure the degree of circular motion that one can make

16

with the distal extremity such as the hand or foot. Rolling inwards is called inversion and eversion is the movement rolling outwards.

For an example with upper body injuries, one can check the range of motion after a shoulder injury by measuring how far up (laterally) one can raise the arm (or raise it by holding into a broom stick as done in picture #13, (page 54.) Then measure how far forwards and backwards one can move the arm, and keep these records for comparison with ROM tests after a few weeks.

• Strength

For *strength testing*, you should measure this in a repeatable way that measures exactly your maximum strength *before pain erupts.* For a knee injury, you could measure your strength to fully extend your knee with a straight leg raise, (Picture #39, page 86). If you can do that without pain, then measure that while using a light ankle weight.

• Endurance

For testing endurance, see how many times you can perform your initial exercise before your joint feels fatigued. (For the initial exercise see the clinical protocols in Chapter IV.) If you do not have exercise testing fatigue after more than 100 repetitions, then test with cardiovascular equipment. It is very important to record the conditions for your test, so take note of the same seat height, the program selected, and the resistance, so that when you repeat the test at a later time, you will be effectively testing *apples vs. apples.*

For the knee injury, you can measure your time on an ergonomic, stationary bicycle with a certain, measured resistance level. (A good instrument for your testing and further training is the Life Fitness, Lifecycle ® because it has the best biomechanical alignment with the best programs for random-resistance and interval training). For injuries to the upper extremities, if you have no fatigue with multiple repetitions of your initial strength test, then you can use arm ergonometry equipment, which allows your arms to make cyclical movement and many gyms and fitness centers have this equipment, such as the SciFit® or Schwin® machines that we use in our wellness center.

Setting Your Rehab Goals

There are four primary tasks you must complete so that you can fulfill your goals in rehabilitation, and your goals should exceed beyond setting your goal as *"Getting better."*

First, ***Write down your ultimate goal.*** [20] Perhaps your goal would be to strengthen the injured knee, so that pain from climbing stairs no longer occurs. You can have many such goals for your rehabilitation, and writing them down will help you measure your progression towards these goals. The goal I mentioned of having no knee pain when climbing stairs is worthwhile but there may also be performance goals that you want for your sport or recreational activity.

The second task is to write down ***How others will know when you have reached your goal.*** [20] Are there people who are helping you deal with your injury such as a spouse? How will they know that you have reached you goal, before you tell them so? Perhaps a performance goal or measurement will accomplish this for you, such as playing four rounds of tennis with no elbow pain, or climbing stairs for 10 minutes.

Third, list the ***things that you can accomplish along the rehab pathway to your final goals.*** To help track your efforts, you should use a ***Progress Chart.*** For example, I kept progress charts during the three, long years of each of the 16 operations, because progress would have been difficult to follow because the operation sequence was: operation – rehab – recovery – operation – rehab, etc. It could have been easy to think that I was not getting anywhere, but because I was using a *Progress chart* after each operation I clearly saw and enjoyed my progress! So if your rehab goal is to climb stairs without pain after knee rehab, then plan to track when you can climb 10 without pain, 25, 50, and 75 stairs without pain. That is better than just setting the goal of climbing to the top of the Empire State Building because you need smaller goals that will help you progress towards the top goal.

Progress Charting

A progress chart is what is used in medical and physical therapy clinics. Having a notebook to track what you have done in the gym is valuable for bodybuilding to knee rehab, so make it a tool that you use. This will help you see progress in both endurance and strength training. Make a chart for each week, and then you will insert the exercise and variables that you use to design your rehab phases in the clinical examples in Chapter IV. One could look like this.

Week One Day one	Angle ROM	Strength test (After your pain abates)	Endurance	Weekly Pain Test
	90° flexion before pain	SLR with 5lbs	10 reps with 5 lbs	35 of 110
Day three	80° flexion before pain	SLR with 5lbs	12 reps with 5lbs	Test weekly
Days 5 and 7	Note changes		Changes?	
Week two	Add other exercises →			Pain test score was 30 of 110

Long Range Goals

It might be easier to set your long-term goals first, and then you can determine the steps needed to reach that ultimate rehab goal. For example, with an ankle fusion the ultimate goal is to secure the bones into a cohesive, strong, stable orthopedic structure that allows the patient to walk and stand without pain. This type fusion procedure normally requires a year of recovery time for complete fusion, but even with a persistent bone infection that is frequently fatal, my rehab recovery was faster than expected. My surgeons said that it was because of my commitment and adherence to my gradual progression through the rehab steps and phases.

After setting the long-term goal then one should set small goals to reach the final destination. Whether your injury was of bone, muscle, or connective tissue (ligaments and tendons), one must remember that it takes time for bones deposition to occur and sometimes even more time for connective tissue recovery. One small goal in rehabilitating my ankle after the fusion operations was to return to indoor cycling. I had many accomplishments that I had to do before that such as "friction weight bearing" for two weeks, but the cycling was a small goal towards my long-range goal of returning to competitive athletics and flying aerobatic planes again.

Short-term goals

A beginning short-term goal might be to regain free movement. Consulting physical therapists will help you with this, and it can be particularly important for your complete recovery. With leg injuries, learning the proper techniques for the safe use of a walker, or crutches, or even a cane, can really benefit you because improper use can injure you. Using these tools when needed will enhance and make your rehab recovery as fast as possible. In my case, I was in a wheelchair for most of the first nine months after the plane crash.

The times when I started using a walker in physical therapy was very exciting and empowering (even though I was in full-leg casts). I used to enjoy conversing with my PT about how many times I would circle the entire hospital building for each session of training with a walker or crutches. This type of exercise can also be effective as strength training. I needed to increase my strength and endurance so that I could abandon my need for a wheelchair as soon as the casts were removed.

Once your healthcare provider has informed you that weight bearing or more movement can be attempted, then you can pursue the next small goal or movement. In my case when I was allowed to start bearing weight on my foot/ankle it was just "friction contact" with the ground at first. Then I was able to bear only percentages of full weight while I was supporting my movement with crutches. It is a fine line but being able to push yourself without going to far, while working hard in your rehab will pay off. Good, frequent communication with one's health care provider will help you find such success in acute injuries or even with a sprained ankle.

Regardless what your injury was, you must always remember that progression is a pathway, not an instantaneous change. I accomplished my weight bearing in the morning before I was fatigued and felt too much pain. This allowed me to keep from becoming over-fatigued, so proceeding this way helped me alleviate the need for most pain medication. It will help you to work with as little pain medication as possible because taking pain-meds will also inhibit bone deposition. So taking less pain medication could mean a faster recovery.

One may now become anxious and impatient while asking yourself, "How or when will I accomplish full recovery." The answer to this question can be found in your progression down the pathway of different rehab *Phases.* You can find success and progression when you accomplish a rehab exercise without pain today, which was painful just 3 days ago. Use a calendar with your *Progress Chart* to record your progression, and after a few weeks you can make an estimate on the time you'll need to complete your rehab.

Chapter III
Determine the Components for Rehab Success

Flexibility is an integral component both for rehabilitation and for all activities and/or exercise. The definition of flexibility training or stretching is to gain maximum extension and flexion of joints in manners that achieve the maximum range of motion. While it is easy for most people to understand why they should regain the muscle strength, many may not recognize the importance in flexibility training.

Flexibility Training

The following are key benefits of flexibility training and stretching:
- Increase Range of Motion (ROM)
- Muscle relaxation for freer movement with less pain
- Increased capacity for venous blood flow, thereby increasing circulation
- It is also a way of preparing the body for exercise or activity, and in this way it is like a signal to prepare muscle for activation
- Reduction of stress

Stretching Techniques and Methods

The blanket rule or technique of stretching is to hold each stretch repetition, for 20 – 30 seconds where there is constant muscle tension. One should not try to pull too tightly because that can cause micro tears, and you should definitely avoid "Bouncing" which can also cause significant tears of the muscle, connective tissues, and cross bridge muscle fibers of the muscle.

There are four main stretching techniques and different techniques follow different rehabilitation phases.

22

• *Passive, Static stretching* is a technique that uses gravity and/or position to gain the effect of gently stretching one's muscle fibers. This can best be described with the stretching of an elbow. The elbow is positioned, outstretched on a table (palm up) with one's wrist and forearm being pressed down only by gravity. (See picture #24 and 25, page 65.) Such a stretch is appropriate in the *Acute phase* of treating Tennis Elbow.

• *Primary Stretching* uses the techniques of obtaining muscle tension and holding it for 20 to 30 seconds, by using the opposing muscle (antagonist) or positioning to achieve the tension for stretching. This is the technique most often used in sports medicine training, (see picture #32, page78). For example a "groin stretch" where one sits with feet together, leaning forward, and uses the body position to make the groin (gracilius) muscle tense.

• *Primary Assisted Stretching* uses force of another person to achieve additional muscle tension. ∇ This technique should only be done with a trained physical therapist, athletic trainer, or a trained physician, because it can easily result in compounding the injury being treated. [1,2,8,15,16] An example of primary assisted stretching is for the hamstring, where one lays with his back on the ground (supine), and a partner raises one of the athlete's legs for extra tension.

• *Proprioceptive Neuromuscular Facilitation* (PNF) is the stretching used for increased force production in athletics. In this strength training technique, one stretches one muscle group intensely before performing a forceful contraction of that muscle group, and this technique is only appropriate in the *Recovery phase* of rehabilitation or for advanced exercise training. An example of PNF, is the Jump Squat used by high-jump athletes, right before their jump over the bar. In this example PNF is similar to Plyometric training that will be discussed later in this chapter.

Stretching, just like strength training, must advance gradually, and this can be done by using changes in the Frequency, Intensity and Time or duration (*F.I.*T). This allows subtle variations for gradual progression, rather than just increasing the intensity of the stretch. *FIT* is another integral component of complete rehabilitation, and utilization of *F.I.T* changes will be described with clinical examples, starting in

23

chapter IV, and it will also be discussed in chapter V, regarding design of your rehabilitation program.

Stretches for each body region

All of the stretch exercises have different benefits, and each stretch is appropriate for a specific *Phase* in your rehabilitation. The following is a large list of important stretches, and you should use this list in choosing options and variations for your *Recovery phase* training. Doing some stretches out of sequence may cause further injuries. Use this list after you have read over the existing rehab programs, listed in chapter IV.

NECK/UPPER BACK
    Range of Motion (ROM)
    Head Rotation
    Passive, Static Stretching
    Self Hug
    Sternocleidomastoid-Trapezius stretch
    Knee Tuck
    Illiopsoas stretch
    Arm extended Cervical ROM
    Reverse incline neck crunch
    Hanging Bend over stretch

LOWER BACK
    Range of Motion (ROM)
    "Tummy Bridging" stretch
    Hamstring stretching
    Back extension
    Elongation stretches
    Seated Trunk twist (shoulder to opposite knee)
    Reverse crunch
    Max squat stretch (butt to heels)
    Side bend stretch
    Lie supine and unilateral knee abduction stretch
    Standing forward flexion

SHOULDERS
    Range of Motion (ROM)
    Shoulder Stretch (hands apart)
    Scapula Stretch (hands together)
    Lying elbow abduction/adduction
    Plyometric Lower Medicine Ball swinging/catch
    Shrug stretch
    Two handed towel behind back

UPPER ARM/ELBOW
    Range of Motion (ROM)
    Passive, Static Elbow Stretching
    Biceps Flexion stretch (with rotation to stretch both
    biceps heads)
    Triceps stretching

LOWER ARM/WRIST
    Range of Motion (ROM)
    Passive, Static Stretching
    Wrist flexor stretch
    Wrist extensor stretch
    Shoulder across stretch
    Praying palm-to-palm stretch
    Waiter's Tip stretch

HIP/THIGH
    Range of Motion (ROM)
    Supine Knee Tuck
    Abductor Groin stretch
    Supine Piriformis stretch
    Hamstring stretches
    Medial Quadriceps stretch
    Lateral Quadriceps stretch
    Illiopsoas stretch
    Standing forward flexion
    Step-Up Lunge stretch
    Standing, Leg elevated to side and bend to side

KNEE
    Range of Motion (ROM)
    Passive Knee Flexion & stretching

Quadriceps stretching (medial and lateral)
Passive Knee Flexion & stretching
Cycle for ROM
Gracilius/Groin stretches
Distal Quad stretch, (lie supine and pull/slide heel towards the gluteus)

LOWER LEG

Ankle Range of Motion (ROM) for co-activation of lower leg muscles
Runner's calf muscle stretch (foot in neutral, open, and closed positions)
Towel calf stretch
Max squat stretch (butt to heels)

FOOT/ANKLE

Range of Motion (ROM)
Foot flexion (in linear motion)
Foot extension
Inversion/Eversion stretching
Rotation Stretching
Dorsi flexion stretching
Plantar flexion stretching
Calf muscle stretching
Stretching plantar fascia (While seated, place your bare foot over a rolling pin that is
upon a hard floor. Then roll the sole of your foot over the rolling pin.)
Rotation ROM
Max squat stretch (butt to heels)

Components of Strength Training

The primary goal in strength training is to increase the number of muscle fibers firing or increase the rate at which the muscle fibers fire. A more powerful muscle contraction may stress the muscle, (without injury), and the body's response is to build towards muscle hypertrophy.

Muscle hypertrophy is gain in the diameter of the muscle fibers, which results in more powerful contractions. Increase in the number of skeletal muscle fibers is hyperplasia, but unfortunately this is not possible in human skeletal muscle. Blood supply is needed for repair of the injured tissue and exercise increases the blood flow to the muscular tissues by up to 25-times greater amounts. [24]

In rehabilitation we want to achieve both increased motor unit activation and increases in the muscles' size, because muscle atrophy is commonly a large factor in many orthopedic injuries such as knee disorders. [2,3,6,11,12] These two gains can be accomplished in unison with the proper rehabilitation *phase* progression.

For example with a knee injury, one can increase the number of muscle fibers firing by training the knee extension with different biomechanical changes in positioning, (such as straight leg raises with straight foot position vs. an open, plie' foot alignment). Then one can obtain hypertrophy (increased muscle size) of the knee muscle by utilizing the Open Stance Cycling Protocol that preferentially activates and trains the medial knee muscle (VMO).

The different type of muscle fiber being trained should be an important component to consider in rehabilitation. There are three primary types of muscle they include: cardiac, smooth muscle (like in the intestines), and striated, skeletal muscle. The skeletal muscle is made up of different fiber types: fast twitch fibers (which are used for instant strength contractions such as weight lifting), and slow twitch fibers for endurance activities such as marathons and postural control.

The collection of different fibers are found in most all muscles, and the fiber type and number can not be changed, but a certain fiber type may be trained for greater, more effective activation. This is why some people have a genotype that makes them better at power muscle exercise (fast twitch) vs. some people who are better at endurance exercises with slow twitch muscle activation. [1,2,22]

Three things are measured in science to differentiate between these fiber types, and they are: Contractile functioning (speed and force of contraction), Morphology (how they look, or appear), and Biochemical sensitivity. The Fast Twitch fibers can have a contraction that happens 4 times faster than the slow twitch fibers, and this ability is linked to the speed at which the electro-chemical signal is transmitted through the muscles. Fast twitch muscles also fire without the need for extra oxygen for the energy of their contractions, hence exercises involving fast twitch muscle activation are often called "anaerobic." Slow twitch fibers have a slower contraction linked with a greater resilience, and their contractions use high amounts of oxygen in the transfer of energy to fuel the contractions. This is called aerobic muscle activation.

The morphology of these type fibers (the different appearance) includes having different colors and they vary in shape. Slow twitch are more red due to the increased oxygen and different shape, and fast twitch fibers are larger in diameter for more powerful, instant contractions. The NFL running back Marcus Allen would have more fast twitch muscle fibers for his sprints requiring instant speed, compared to Steve Prefontaine who had more slow twitch fibers active as a top endurance, Olympic runner of the seventies.

Exercises for Strength Training

This is a large, list of the important exercises for each body region, but this list is to show you the options that you may choose from in designing your continued *Recovery phase* training. Exercises in rehabilitation are phase dependant, and there are times that they would be beneficial and times that the same exercise would injure you. Use this list to choose exercises for variation in the *Recovery phase* of your rehab training.

NECK/UPPER BACK
Isometric muscle activation
Isotonic contraction against immoveable object
Wall Press

Latissimus Dorsi cable rows
"Shrug" Trap Lifts
Seated Rhomboid row (flat grip or hammer grip)
Prone, single dumbbell row
Dips
Swimming

LOWER BACK

Spider Crawl exercise (free or with weights)
Straight Leg Raise (SLR)
Isotonic contraction against immoveable object
Abdominal "Crunches"
Supine "Marching" legs
Pelvic tilt
Incline Rows
Seated Rows
Oblique Crunches
Hyperextension lifts
Seated twists
Incline leg raises
Hanging knee-raises
Wall Squats

SHOULDERS

Pendulum Control
Wall Presses
Plyometric Lower Medicine Ball swinging/catch
Butterfly Elbow Abduction (free, with weights, or on a machine)
Rope Pulley
Ball on Wall movements
Isometric biceps curls
Triceps extensions
T-Bar row
Cycling machine
Seated rowing machine
Glenohumoral extension
Bar press
Supine Karate chop exercises

Curl bar row
Latissimus Dorsi Pull down (to chest or to back)
Incline Dumbbell pres
Abduction cable row (single handed grips)
Dumbbell curls behind back (with arms fully extended)

UPPER ARM/ELBOW
Biceps flexion/rotation
Stick rotation
Hammer rotation
Overhead Medicine Ball Movement
Opposite stick and Hammer
Medicine Ball swing
Wind Up weight
Isometric joystick movements
Dumbbell Butterfly exercise
Towel twist
Cable press down
Hammer curls
Rotation curls

LOWER ARM/WRIST
Wrist Flexion (isometric or weighted)
Wrist Extension (isometric or weighted)
Hammer rotation
Dumbbell balance overhead
Towel twist
Pushing against a wall
Rope Pulley
Power grip
Grip & Pull
Tennis ball squeeze
Volleyball on wall
Wrist Curl
Reverse curl

HIP/THIGH
Pillow compression between knees
Standing on one leg (with extra isometric contractions)
Leg abduction with weight

Leg Slide (extension exercise)
Squats (Smith Machine® for stability)
Leg adduction (elastic band resistance)
Skiing machines
Seated Knee Abduction/Adduction machine
Leg Extension machine (Incline or flat)
Hip Flexor band exercise
Supine marching
Aquatic therapy (freestyle kick or frog kick)
Hamstring curls (prone or seated)
Standing Knee to Chest exercise
Hanging knee-raises
Lunges
Wall squats

KNEE

Straight leg Raise
Stationary Bicycle training
Open Stance Cycling protocol
Smith Squats
Side Walking (with weights)
Cycle for ROM completion
Sled knee extension
Individual knee extension machine exercise
Seated Knee curl
Prone hamstring curl
Hanging repeated knee raises
Knee extension "Holds" at 120 degrees on machine

LOWER LEG

Isometric contractions (anterior tibialis)
Foot Extension exercise
Elliptical Machine exercise
Non-impact cardiovascular training
Seated calf raises

FOOT/ANKLE

Cable resistance for plantar flexion
Cable resistance for dorsi flexion
Isometric contractions

Straight leg raise
Line Jumping
Foot-board exercises
Smith Squats
Jumping in swimming pool (no foot impact upon landing)
Stationary Cycling
Single Leg stance
Alternating heel raise
Plantar flexion against towel
Dorsi flexion against towel
Lunges

Plyometric Exercises

Athletes who participate in sports that require instant, maximum power muscle contractions such as football, high jumping, basketball and volleyball often use Plyometric training. Plyometrics could be effective in your final *Recovery phase* of rehabilitation and/or continued training. Plyometric muscle activation begins with a movement that maximally stretches the primary muscle, just before that muscle is contracted. In high jump, the athlete runs towards the bar/platform and first jumps into a deep squat (max quadriceps stretch), before a maximum contraction of those quadriceps muscle fibers propels him over the high bar, and this is a plyometric technique.

The muscles natural recoil ability is involved in plyometric training, and people often train with the "drop jump" described for high jumpers or with "multiple jumps" in basketball, so that they have the best effort when competing. An exercise that uses plyometric training on a small scale is walking with "lunges," and this will be discussed in chapter IV under leg injuries. The research on Plyometrics though has not been adequate, and there is significant potential to damage the musculoskeletal tissue with over-load in Plyometrics. Be cautious in using plyometric exercises because "too much too fast" is almost guaranteed to injure you or disrupt your rehab.

Aerobic, Cardiovascular Training

True cardiovascular, aerobic exercise requires a consistent, steady, elevated heart rate of 70% to 75% of one's maximum heart rate (this is often called a "steady-rate" heart beat). It is called "aerobic" because in this type of endurance exercise, the body requires increased oxygen consumption for energy in this exercise. The cardiovascular training with the "steady-rate" heart beat, has to provide larger amounts of oxygen to the working muscles, and cardiovascular efficiency. A good example of optimal cardiovascular efficiency are those athletes who are able to participate in the 658 mile *Ultra-marathons* where they run 118 miles a day for 5½ days straight.

The oxygen is used in aerobic exercise to help break down the body's fats (lipids such as triglycerides and free fatty acids) for fuel. So a side benefit of aerobic training is an eventual decrease in one's subcutaneous body fat. This exercise regime is effective in weight loss, which is part of why aerobic exercise training is effective in the treatment of Type II Diabetes. (See Chapter VII for further discussion of treating illnesses with exercise.)

Many different exercise modes may be used to achieve this "steady-rate" heart beat, and they include the following:
- Bicycling
- Slow Running or Jogging
- Swimming
- Dancing
- Cross country skiing
- Speed walking
- Ergonomic cycling (leg or arm action)
- Elliptical machine training
- Stair climbing (or Stairmaster machines)
- Treadmills
- Rowing machines
- Cross-robics machines
- Cross training

Like all exercise modes there are different risks with each of these aerobic exercises, and you should decide which is better for your goals based on the risks and fatigue of the muscles being trained. Contemplate how each exercise could effect your injured area and also think about what exercise mode is best for your lifestyle.

For example with all of the outdoor modes, one must be aware that training in congested areas with many motorized vehicles is both dangerous and counter productive because the extra carbon monoxide that cars are emitting deters your ability to consume oxygen from the air you breathe in. So choose a training mode that fits your needs and your environment.

Some of these exercises have risks or cause problems for people with certain injuries. For example, using a stair climbing machine would not be advisable for a person with knee injuries not only because pain from stair climbing often causes pain in injured knees, but also because the shear force on the knee cap (patella) when pressing down the step pedal can worsen the injury. The risks and precautionary information is provided in the sections of Chapter IV.

Aerobic, cardiovascular training has many great benefits and uses, even for athletes who participate in anaerobic sports such as weight lifting and sprint running, and the use of this type training for different, common injuries will be discussed more fully, in the clinical perspectives of Exercise Therapy in Chapter IV.

Prayer and Spiritual Therapy

In the components for rehab success have you considered asking God for help? After being injured, many people may feel "Mad at God", but both my experience and clinical medical testing has shown that prayer does aid in recuperation and healing, (even if the prayers come from people other than the patient). 36

Perhaps one might call on the greatest Teacher and Healer of all time for help, and that is God. My accident was one of the most traumatic imaginable, but rather than being mad, I was joyous and thanking God many times each day that I was alive and had another chance – at everything! Still today, more than a dozen years after my crash, I still thank God for His healing, care, and for who His influence who has made me who I am today.

The best thing is that with God, "Anything is possible." [37] One only has to ask for God's help and then accept His grace and unconditional love. Listen for His whispers of advice; confirm His intentions in the Bible, and then "Press on" towards His goals for you.

Chapter IV
Exercise Therapy, Upper Extremities and Upper Torso

This chapter will reveal exercises therapy programs that have been designed to treat the common, orthopedic injuries of the upper torso and upper extremities. Examining the current exercise therapies is the fourth step for complete recovery and recuperation, but it may be the most physically and emotionally challenging *step* because it is not like a light switch that can be turned on. However, sticking to the *Steps* and Phases of training described in this book will make your rehab effective, efficient, and lasting.

The exercise therapy for complete rehabilitation will take some time, and with this in mind, one may ask the question "Why is rehabilitation of common, non-traumatic injuries necessary?" The answer begins with the need to resolve the symptomatic problems. For example if one has chronic or frequent tennis elbow (Lateral Epicondylitis), there may have been a muscle weakness or muscular asymmetry that caused reoccurrence of the painful symptoms. If the injury is treated with appropriate rehabilitative training, the weakness will be overcome and the tendonitis (inflammation of tendons) should not reoccur. 2

Goals of Rehabilitation

The techniques and steps to be utilized in effective orthopedic rehabilitation will be focused on the following priorities: 1) Decreasing the symptoms, 2) Regaining complete range of motion (ROM), 3) Neuromuscular Control, 4) Flexibility training, and 5) Strength training. This will allow one to return to the pre-injury state and regain that level of performance in his/her sport or activity. If this is not done, the injured person may suffer from muscle atrophy (loss of muscle size and strength), and the decreased muscle fiber diameters will result in weakness, and decreased muscular endurance. If one chooses

36

to treat an orthopedic injury with inactivity, it could yield significant muscle atrophy. Such inactivity could decrease the muscle mass by up to 40% in just three weeks. [1]

Rehabilitation will also help one restore fitness for other activities, including cardiovascular efficiency. It has also been shown that one's cardiovascular fitness and efficiency can also be reduced by up to 25% after three weeks of only treating an injury with rest. [2]

Stair-Steps Goals of Rehabilitation
1. Reduced pain, inflammation, and swelling
2. Healing of the tissue
3. Regain the joint's range of motion, (ROM)
4. Restore complete neuromuscular control of the injured area
5. Counteract the tendency for muscle atrophy
6. Regain and increase strength and power
7. Reactivate and ensure proprioceptive abilities, (sensation of muscle contraction), and
8. Regain and increase endurance for sport and normal activities

The list of goals above may seem large but rehabilitation works to accomplish all of these goals by progressively achieving "Stair steps" of progression. The steps will be achieved by following specific training phases that are common in treating all different orthopedic disorders, and the phases are: The Acute phase, Rehab phase, and the Recovery phase. These phases were described in detail in the Introduction, and the table below shows an overview of the rehab phases.

<u>Overview of Phases</u>

Acute Phase: FIRST 3 DAYS
R.I.C.E.
Passive, Static stretching
ROM

Rehab Phase: DAY 4 to 14
Flexibility training
Neuromuscular training
Light resistance

Recovery: WEEKS 3 to 6
Flexibility
Progressive resistance
Proprioceptive training

Rehab Progression and *F.I.T.*

The method for altering the protocol to achieve progress is *F.I.T.,* which stands for changing the Frequency, Intensity and Time or duration in exercise. This allows for more subtle variations of gradual progression, rather than just increasing the resistance (Intensity) or time exercising. *FIT* is another integral component of Stair Step progression. Examples of this will be shown in exercise therapies for specific, common injuries.

Exercise Therapies
This section will address the regions of the upper torso and upper extremities, and this section will include therapeutic protocols for common injuries in those areas. It will describe the majority of therapeutic protocols for increasing the ROM, neuromuscular activation, strength training, and then include proactive exercises. Each section will close with a *Rehab summary* of the different protocols to be used in each *phase* of rehabilitation for that injury.

NECK INJURIES

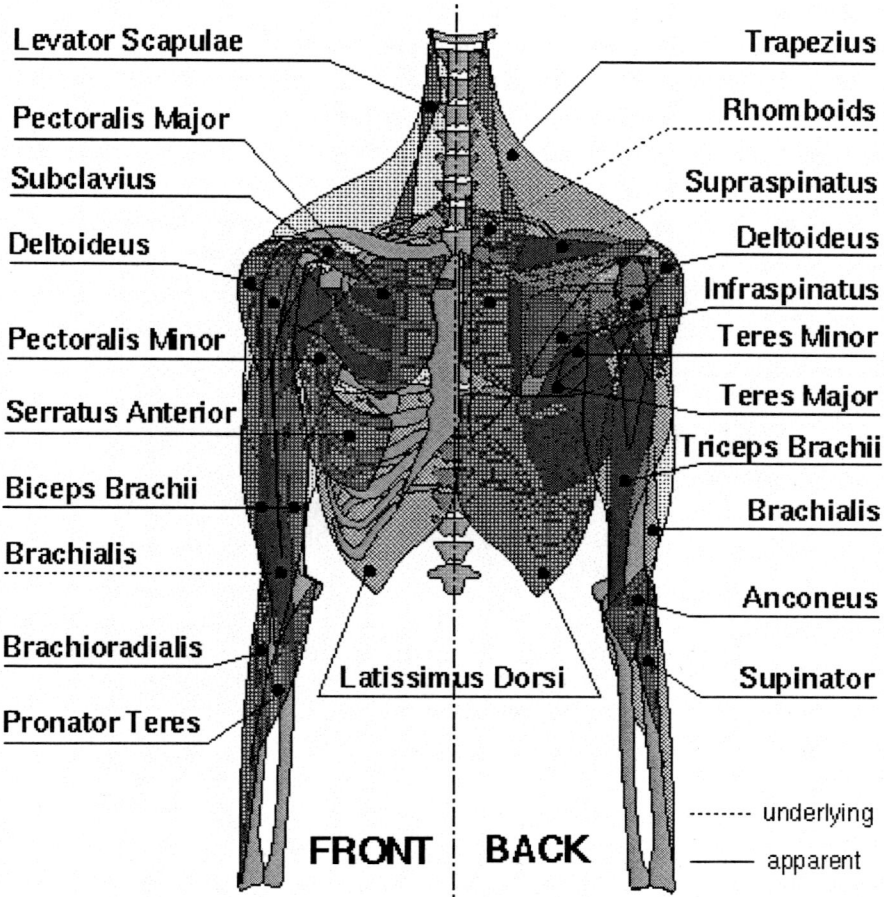

Levator Scapulae

Pectoralis Major

Subclavius

Deltoideus

Pectoralis Minor

Serratus Anterior

Biceps Brachii

Brachialis

Brachioradialis

Pronator Teres

Trapezius

Rhomboids

Supraspinatus

Deltoideus

Infraspinatus

Teres Minor

Teres Major

Triceps Brachii

Brachialis

Anconeus

Supinator

Latissimus Dorsi

FRONT **BACK**

-------- underlying

———— apparent

Figure #1, Upper torso musculature

Cervical strain

This is a common injury acquired from very different settings ranging from racquetball to gymnastics, or contusion, impact injuries in American football. [1] The symptoms include pain on one side of the neck that develops into a continued, dull ache that can often yield sharper pain. Having a stiff neck with muscle spasm are also frequent symptoms.

In the *Acute phase* of treatment one must use *RICE,* plus stretching and possibly light massage. One must begin with

Rest by eliminating stressful exercise and/or painful positioning. Then use Ice packs to help reduce the swelling and inflammation will also help. While using Compression on one's neck is inadvisable, the Elevation while lying in bed or sitting in a reclining chair may help substantially. In this phase one can work on regaining flexibility by using Head Rotation and Passive, Static Stretching.

The head rotation stretch is done by stretching your head at the 12, 3, 6, and 9 o'clock positions, (as if a clock were flat on top of your head). Move your head forward at 12 o'clock until there is light tension and holding that spot for 20 seconds. Then tilt your head to the right side at 3 o'clock until there is tension, and hold the stretch for 20 seconds. Then do similar movement to the 6 and 9 o'clock positions.

The Passive, Static Stretching is where one simply uses gravity to acquire the tension rather than pulling on the extremity or using devices for such movement, and yields a safe stretch for treatment. For the passive, static stretch of the neck, simply tilt the head over and hold a stretch for at least 20 seconds. Avoid the old "bouncing or bobbing" techniques that were used in the past. It is now proven that such bouncing can cause micro, muscle tears, which obviously will not help. [8]

Relaxing massage by a Registered, licensed Massage Therapist can be helpful but make sure to inform the massage therapist what area(s) or movements that are painful, so that manipulation of those areas will be avoided. Sometime the therapist can use traction on a patient's neck while the person is lying on their back, and this can be effective in reducing the pressure on the cervical disks.

The **Rehab phase** can add more exercise and techniques for enhancing neuromuscular control, and beginning strength training. For strength training in the rehab phase, you should only perform isometric muscle activation. Isometric training is to contract the muscle without movement. For example if one puts the forearm and upper arm into a 90-degree position and then simultaneously flexes the biceps and triceps muscles without moving the arm, this would be called isometric muscle contraction.

One can use stable resistance for increased strength training of the neck muscles. To do this, simply lean your head onto your hand, and push your head against your hand without allowing any movement.

The ***Recovery phase*** will focus on gradually returning to the activities and the sports participated in, before the injury. Design a plan that prescribes exercise for every other day, and change one of *FIT* (Frequency, Intensity or Time training), once each week. Rotational clock-stretching (described on the previous page), is an effective technique, and can be done as a proactive treatment to prevent pain from erupting, (i.e. if one has to ride in a car along a bumpy road or sit still for an extended amount of time).

Additional strength training in this phase can include the shrug exercise. In this exercise one starts in an upright position and lifts the shoulders without raising the arms. This can later be made more challenging by holding dumbbells while the shrug is performed. (See picture #2.)

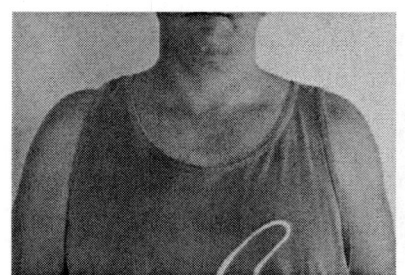
Pic #2 Pre Shrug

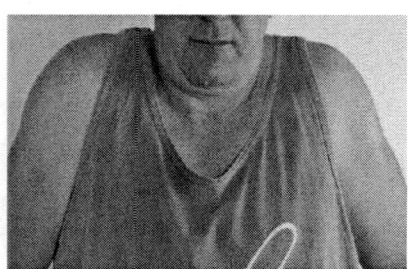
Pic #2 Trap Shrug

Cervical Strain Rehab summary
Acute Phase: FIRST 3 DAYS
R.I.C.E.
Passive, Static stretching
Relaxing light massage
Rehab Phase: DAY 4 to SECOND WEEK
Passive, Static Stretching
Isometric muscle contraction
Stable resistance
Recovery: WEEKS 3 to 6
Proactive Stretching
Shrug Exercises

Neck Tension

Neck tension and tension headaches are a frequent problem for many people, and it may be effectively treated with exercises for increased flexibility and increased blood flow to the orthopedic structures in that region. The most obvious symptom is a stiff neck but frequently this condition also includes muscle spasm and continued muscle tension (muscle tetany).

In the *Acute phase* the treatment is similar to that of the cervical strain in using ice packs with passive, static stretching and light massage. Rest will be an important component to this phase because one must ensure that the condition does not worsen. It should be important to rule out neck disorders that can be more serious and require immediate medical care. Eliminate the following conditions before proceeding with exercise therapy:

* Congenital Torticolis or a *Wry neck,* is a condition often confused with chronic neck strain, and this condition can contain small fibrous tumors and is a chronic condition. To determine if this condition has occurred, ask yourself if the neck is always in a unusual, fixed position. If the answer is "Yes" then seek medical treatment.

* Injury to Suprascapular Nerve happens when the scapula or collarbone is severely injured or fractured, which results in neck inability to laterally rotate the head, as if the muscles are "blocked." Another symptom of this injury is continual flexion of the wrist, called the "waiter's tip" position. If you have experienced this symptom you must seek immediate medical care.

The *Rehab phase* will focus on flexibility. Utilize further stretching exercises for this phase, and this will include a Sternocleidomastoid-Trapezius stretch and a Self Hug Stretch. [4] (Picture # 3 and #4.) The benefit of flexibility training is that it increases ROM, reduces tension of the muscles, ligaments, and tendons, and it increases venous blood flow. One may also benefit from a deeper tissue massage at this phase. Massage may also help eliminate lactic acid buildups from previous strenuous exercise or activity and enhances the blood flow.

The *Recovery* phase will include the proactive exercises to diminish the occurrence of these symptoms of this condition. Adding to the flexibility training one will need to add stationary cardiovascular (CV) training that will help increase blood flow to areas with poor vascular enervation. A good piece of equipment for this exercise could include a Lifecycle® stationary bicycle or Stair Master® machine. Running may jar the injured area rather than assisting in the recovery.

Neck Tension Rehab summary

Acute phase:	RICE
	Eliminate other disorders
	Light Massage
	Passive, Static Stretching
Rehab phase:	4 Additional Stretches
	Deeper Massage
Recovery	Continued stretching
	Stationary CV training

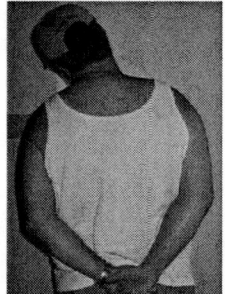
Pic #3 Sterno-Trap stretch

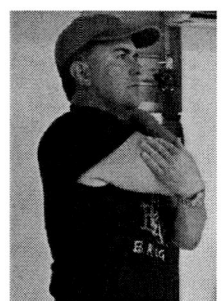
Pic #4 Self Hug stretch

Additional training for neck injuries can include doing neck (cervical) range of motion while lying on one arm extended, (Picture #5). To do this one will lie on their side with one arm extended beneath the head. Then move the head in up and down motions and in rotation to strengthen the neck.

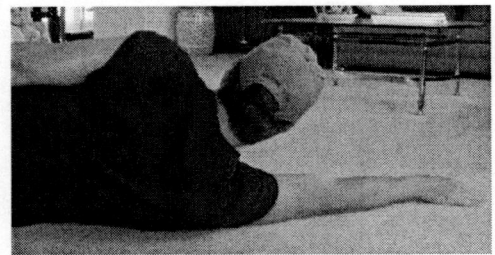

Pic #5 Cervical ROM

BACK INJURIES

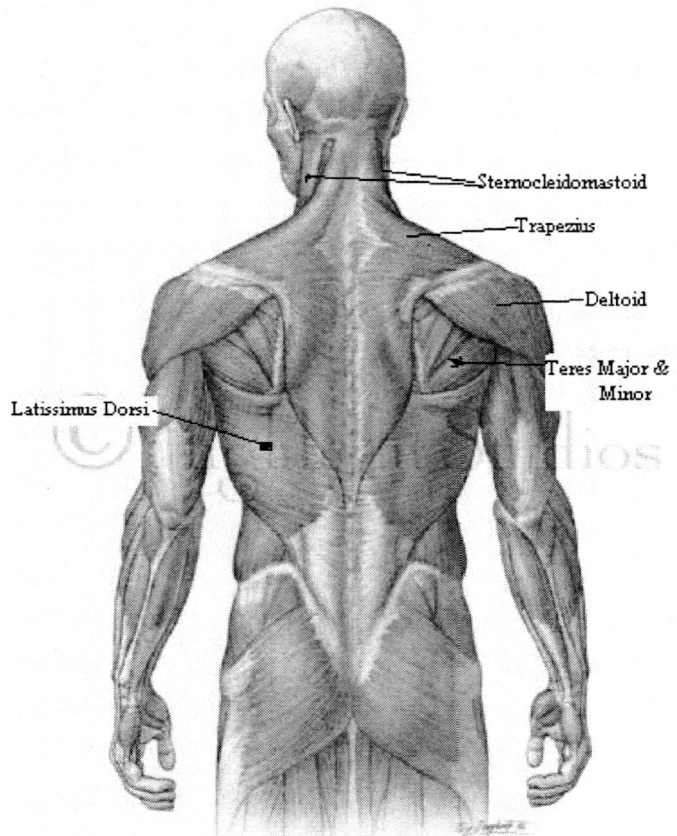

Figure #2, Scapular Back Illustration

Thoracic, Scapular Muscle Strain

This type of injury can come from overuse, such as with golf or contact injuries such as soccer or basketball, or this injury could occur from heavy weight lifting movements. Symptoms that are seen with this injury include a sudden "pull" and/or a sharp pain in the back. Frequently the pain may subside in a few hours, and an athlete may return to his/her activity but the pain will later erupt more severely. If pain radiates down the limbs, then one should immediately consult a physician to ensure that a neural injury has not occurred.

The *Acute phase* again first uses *RICE*, and the Rest from such exercise or activity should be mandated for at least one week because if this injury is not treated it can later cause painful problems from the neck to the lower back. Ice packs are effective, and Compression may be needed depending on the severity of the injury. If compression is needed then medical attention should be acquired. Elevation can be achieved on one's bed by elevating the head section of the mattress with bricks under that part of the bed frame. An effective stretching technique to use is the Self Hug.

For the Self Hug, simply stand and place your right hand over your left shoulder and then place your left hand over the right shoulder. Simply contract your arm muscles, which will stretch the back muscles in opposition. (Picture #5.)

Upon starting the *Rehab phase* one can use the Knee-Tuck stretch. Begin by lying supine, on your back, then simply bend your knees and pull them to your chest. This can be gradually increased as your recovery progresses. A strength training exercise that is effective is the Spider-Extension. (Picture #6.) Start out by being on your hands and knees, and then lift alternating limbs. First lift the right arm and hold it out for 15 seconds and then extend the left leg, holding it in the air for another 15 seconds. Then alternate using the opposite arm and leg in a similar manner.

To make the Spider-Extension more strenuous (as your rehab progresses), you can extend the limbs with greater force but slower speed. Simultaneously extend your arm and opposite leg, and try to reach out further and harder. This will work the thoracic back muscles in an effective manner.

In the *Recovery Phase* one can use more exercises and eventually use fitness equipment for strengthening the lower trapezius, rhomboid, and latissimus dorsi muscles, (see figure #2).

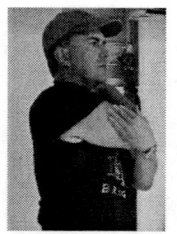

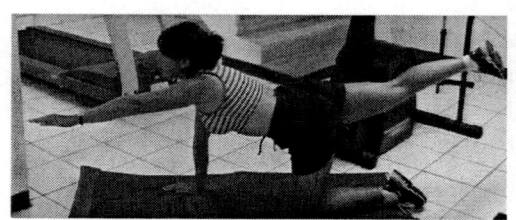

Pic #5, Self Hug　　　　　　　　Pic #6, Spider Extension on knees

An additional stretching technique that is beneficial, is the Knee Across Stretch, also called the Illiopsoas stretch. To accomplish this stretch, lie on your back with one leg extended and one knee flexed to 90 degrees. Then let the flexed knee rotate over the other knee causing tension in the thoracic muscle, and hold the stretch for 20 seconds. (Picture #7.)

Further strength training may begin with a Wall Press also called a runner's stretch. Place your hands on a wall and lean towards the wall. After your elbows are flexed then press away from the wall. (Picture #8.) In the Recovery phase, the Spider-Extension can be made more intense if the starting position is with your stomach on the floor. This position works deeper back muscles and is also used in recovery phase training for lumbar injuries.

The intensity of the wall press exercise is easily increased, by changing the distance of one's feet from the wall until it becomes a regular push-up. Then exercises in the gym or fitness center will help strengthen the weak area to a higher level than before the injury. Common exercises that will help further recovery include the bar pull for latissimus dorsi, seated cable row for the rhomboid muscles (try the 'V' grip handles for variation from the flat bar grip), and free weight rows with the dumbbell pulled to your rib cage is effective too.

Thoracic Strain Rehab summary

Acute phase: R.I.C.E.
Self Hug

Rehab phase: Knee-Tuck Stretch
Spider Extension

Recovery: Wall Press
Intense Spider-Extension
Latissimus Dorsi cable rows

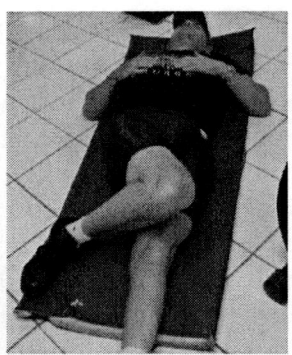

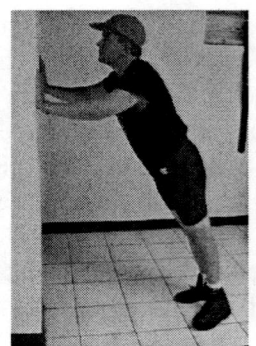

Pic #7, Illiopsoas stretch   **Pic #8** Wall Press

Lumbar, Lower back pain

Lower Back Pain (LBP) is a common condition that affects millions of people, and an estimated 80% of the US population will at some time suffer from lumbar lower back pain. [7] People who have this condition can easily worsen the symptoms with injury to the deep back muscles, which are the Supraspinatus, Erector Spinae, Transverse Spinalis, and Psoas muscles, if they do not seek rehabilitative treatment, (see figures #1 and #2). There are multiple neural anomalies that cause chronic low back pain, and if the condition continues one should seek medical treatment for further diagnosis of the specific problem so that a specific treatment plan can be designed. This injury also has sharp pains that may subside after a few hours but later erupt as "deeper, cutting" pain or it could be a continuing, chronic pain.

Acute phase of a lower back injury will be focused on using ice packs, anti-inflammatory medication, (such as ibuprofen), and it should be accompanied by three days of rest. It is easy to complicate with any stressful movement. Lower back injuries can become more problematic with excessive scar tissue so even flexibility will not be used to treat the acute phase of this injury. After the pain has subsided then one may use a heating pad to help elevate the blood flow for increased tissue repair.

After the first three days, one may begin the *Rehab phase* by training flexibility, but only in the pain free areas. This phase will also benefit from light massage that increases the venous (returning) blood flow to the area to enhance the recuperation. A stretching exercise in this phase that is helpful is the "Tummy Bridging" stretch. One lies supine on the floor and arches one's back for the tummy to be at a higher level. This helps stretch the anterior, deep spinal musculature. (Picture #9.) A hamstring stretch is also effective and relieves tension and allows greater venous blood flow to decrease the deeper inflammation.

Once the pain has subsided then one may also begin using aerobic, cardiovascular training with swimming or a stationary bicycle to supply blood for repair of the damaged tissue. Those two exercises are better than jogging because of reduced weight on the lumbar vertebrae. It has also been described that cardiovascular endurance training helps prevent herniated vertebral disks. [14]

One may also begin strength training without weight, by using gravity resistance. A superb exercise is the Spider Crawl exercise. One will lie on the floor, stomach down, and alternately lift opposing foot and arm. (Picture #10.) This accomplishes very effective strength training of the muscle of the lower back and allows great progression. Another effective exercise is simply a Straight Leg Raise, (SLR). Simply sit on a chair and extend your knee and raise one leg. (see picture #39.)

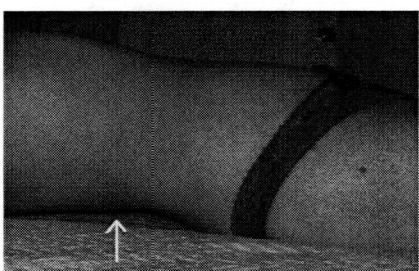

Pic #9 Tummy Bridging
(Note space between lumbar vertebrae & bed)

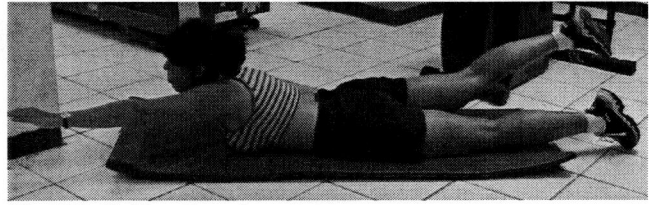

Pic #10, Spider Crawl on tummy

49

In the *Recovery phase* one can use the Spider Crawl for more strenuous training by simultaneously lifting both feet and both arms. This again can use *FIT* to allow progress by timing how long one can hold all limbs off the ground and later use an Intensity change of using ankle weights and light dumbbells (2 pound dumbbells). This phase may also utilize different exercises and stretches for proactive treatment.

An effective proactive exercise to avoid LBP is to start your morning with abdominal "Crunches." Activation of the abdominal muscles helps strengthen the lower torso, which can help reduce the weight and load on your lower back. Another proactive exercise is to simply lie on your back and "March" your legs. Try and extend your legs as far as possible and then also pull your knees up to your chest for effective muscle activation. Once pain has disappeared then one may also start strengthening the lower back with several resistance exercises.

Good resistance exercise for the lower back includes the seated rows and incline rows. (Pictures #11 & #12.) The Seated row can be effective for greater lumbar muscle activation, but it must be done cautiously so that it does not aggravate the injury. Begin by grabbing the handles with your knees flexed, and lift the weight off the stack by extending your legs. Then row your arms to your chest with just a slight movement of your back to the posterior position (slightly lean backwards at the end of your row). The incline rows, allow one to rest his chest on an incline platform and row the weight for activation of lumbar and thoracic muscles.

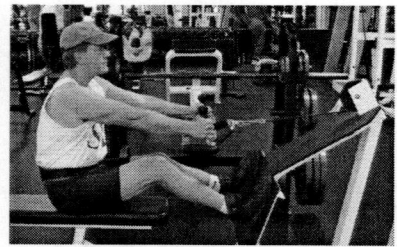
Pic #11 Seated Cable Row: Start

➔

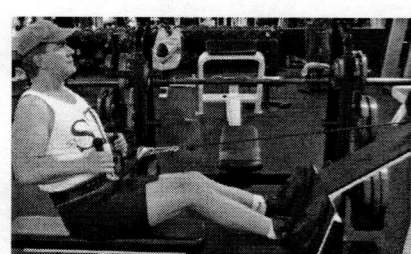
Row Finish

<u>Lower Back Pain Rehab summary</u>
Acute phase: RICE
                        Ibuprofen
                        Heating pad after pain
                            abides
                        NO Exercise or Stretching
Rehab phase: Pain Free Flexibility
                        Hamstring stretch
                        Bridging
                        Stationary bicycling
                        Straight leg raise
Recovery: Crunches
                        Rowing & Spider exercises

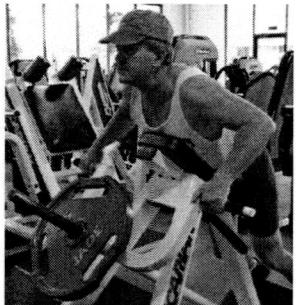

Pic #12 Incline Row

Other strength training exercises for lower back pain include the Pelvic tilt, Oblique Crunches, and Hyperextension lifts. To do the pelvic tilt, simply lie on your back (supine), with you knees bent, and feet and hands on the floor, then elevate you buttocks. Oblique crunches are started by lying on your back and rolling to your side, so that you can "crunch" your shoulder to your hip. Hyperextension lifts are only done in the final stages of *Recovery,* and done on a rack, which holds your legs in a fixed position. Then simply put your fists against your ears without holding onto your head (to avoid cervical injuries), and lower your upper torso followed by raising the upper torso. A unique exercise is a "Reverse Crunch," and this is started by lying on your back. Then smoothly flex your waist and bring your knees to your chest while keeping your legs straight. This action will lift your buttocks off the ground when done properly.

Proactive exercises for lower back pain include performing several different stretches through out the day to prevent back pain and stiffness. Some additional, effective back stretches are: Hamstring stretching, Back Extension stretches, Elongation stretch, Side flexion stretch, and the Supine Transverse stretch (Single flexed knee abduction)

SHOULDER INJURIES

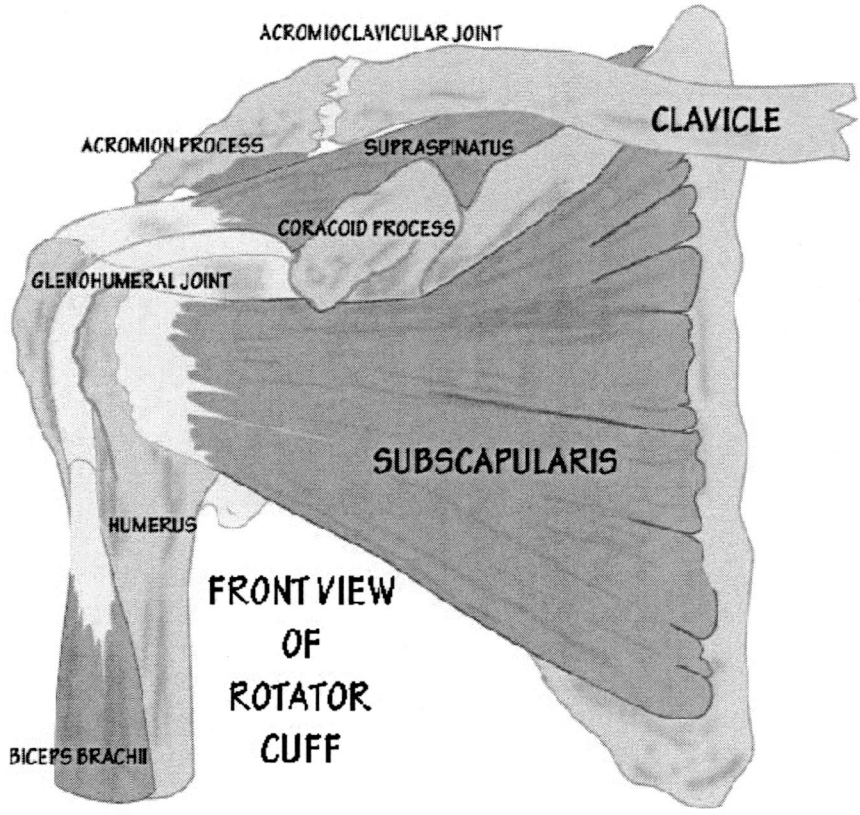

Figure #3, Rotator Cuff musculature, OrthoDoc Massage website

Rotator Cuff Tendonitis

Rotator cuff tendonitis (Supraspinatus tendonitis) is inflammation of the tendon(s) that hold this ball-and-socket joint. The muscular group that cover the compete ball-and-socket joint to the Glenohumeral joint of the shoulder are *SITS:* Supraspinatus, Infraspinatus, Teres Minor, and Subscapularis, as seen in figures #1, #2, and #3. This area is easily injured from many different sports and activities that have repetitive micro traumas from actions such as throwing a baseball with high-intensity, many times (pitcher's shoulder), or it may be caused by repetitively pushing with one's shoulder (as in rugby). Unfortunately these injuries are difficult to completely rehabilitate.

As with most *overuse* injuries, the symptoms can have a gradual onset, and they include the following: pain from elevating the arm between 80° and 120° and tenderness or pain over the Acromion (the bone from the shoulder blade that projects forward through the shoulder girdle).

The **Acute phase** treatment will include rest, ice, and anti-inflammatory medication with little mobility. Cold compression devices may be difficult to find but they are very beneficial in this phase. Try only free movement that is not painful, but always remember that your goal in this *Rehab* phase must be tissue healing. So ensure that all efforts are safe, gradual, pain-free so that you have a protective environment for the tissue to heal.

Regaining ROM and flexibility will be the key goals during the **Rehab phase,** and since there are many different components to rotator cuff tendonitis (many different tendons that could have been injured), strength training will be a slow and very gradual process. The ROM must be trained for pain free elevation of the arm to 90 degrees. (Picture #13.) This can be done by holding onto a broom handle while the other arm pushes up the stick. For an advanced exercise, simply lift your arm to the side, then lower it in front without the assistance of a stick. This will help activate different muscles for rehabilitation.

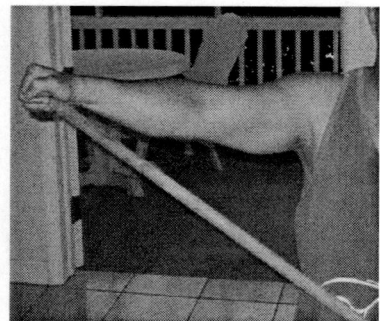
Pic #13, Assisted arm abduction

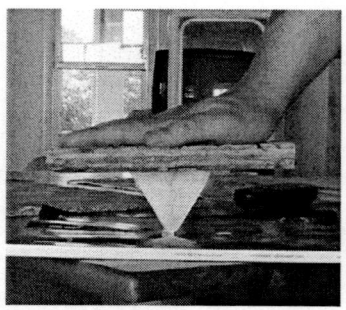
Pic #14 Pendulum

The *Rehab phase* for rotator cuff injuries may be the longest of all injuries because rotator cuff tendonitis is a complex disorder that may require several different exercises for different goals. A good exercise for sensory motor (neural) control is to stand by a table and put one's hands on a pendulum device for controlled oppositional pressure. These devices can be ordered from stores providing supplies for orthopedic injuries such as Allegro Medical supplies.® This is a key exercise for neuromuscular control. (Picture # 14.)

A treatment that enhances ROM, neuromuscular control, and strength training is to use an alternating rope pulley, (Picture #15). This is very effective in contracting both the activator and stabilizer muscles around the deltoid. This helps achieve rehabilitation of the deltoids, supraspinatus, infraspinatus, teres minor, subscapularis, and the tendons & ligaments. A similar movement exercise is to rotate an inflated ball on the wall while standing perpendicular to the wall's surface. This is an effective closed-chained exercise (where the extremity is in weight bearing, fixed contact with a surface), for scapular elevation and depression. (Picture #20.)

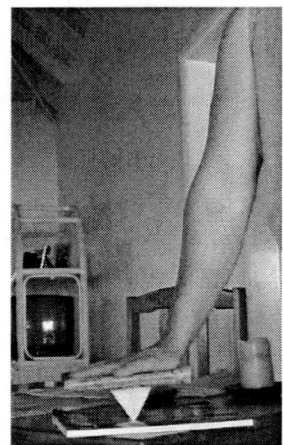

Pic #14-b, Pendulum for NM control

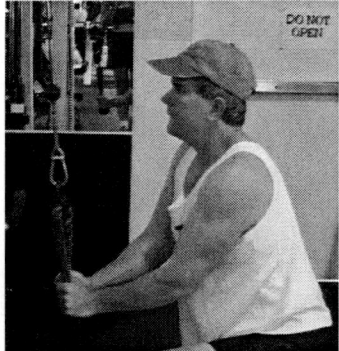

Pic #15 Rope Pulley

After one is pain free and regains significant ROM (beyond the 90 degree arm abduction in unassisted movement), there are very effective exercises in the ***Recovery phase.*** Wall Presses (Picture # 8), are very effective for strengthening the entire rotator cuff muscles and variations for resistance or intensity *FIT* can be made by placing one's feet further from the wall, and changing positions of one's hands can make variations in muscle activity.

Now one can also use Plyometric techniques, which take muscles to the maximum lengthening for increased contraction. Catching, swinging, and throwing a medicine ball with the arms extended is such an exercise. (Picture # 16.) In addition to Plyometric exercises, one might also begin using light dumbbells for an elbow abduction that resembles a butterfly movement. To accomplish the movements for this exercise, pick up a light dumbbell in each hand, bend over slightly, with the elbow contracted to a fixed position of 90 degrees. (Picture # 17.) Then elevate (abduct) the elbows upwards in a muscle action that resembles the butterfly flapping its wings.

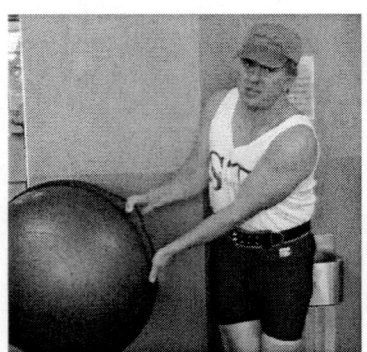 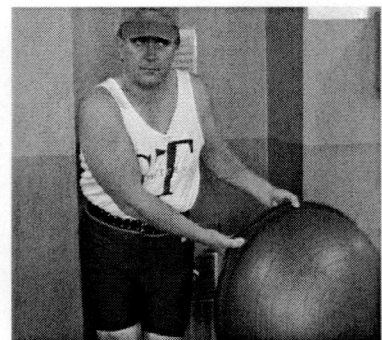

Pic #16 Medicine Ball Swing to   →   Final position

The resistance does not have to increase until one has done different repetitions or sets of the exercise with slow, concentrated motion of both abduction and adduction.

Rotator Cuff Tendonitis Rehab summary
Acute phase: Ice Compression packs
Pain-free movement
Rehab phase: STICK for 90° abduction
Rope Pulley
Ball on Wall movement
Ultrasound
Recovery: Wall Pushups
Butterfly Elbow Abduction
Plyometrics: medicine ball

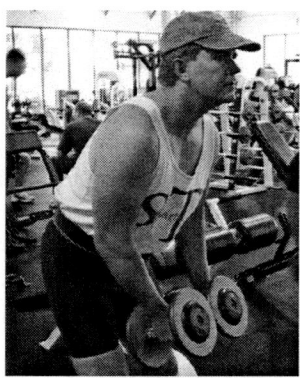 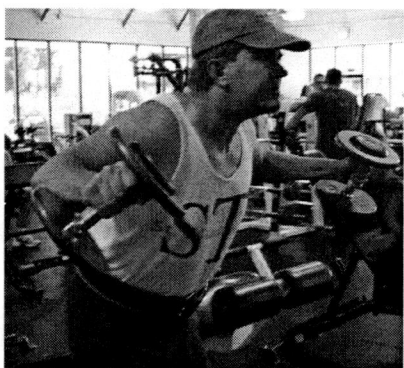

Pic #17 Butterfly BD Abduction start ➔ Finished Contraction

Scapular Injury

The treatment is similar to many of the muscles activated in rehabilitation of rotator cuff tendonitis, but the exercises and changes in *FIT* will be somewhat different. Frequently, scapular injuries are seen with instability of the shoulder's Glenohumoral complex (see figure #3). Symptoms include having an *impingement* to free movement of the arm and one scapula can be "winged" or protruding from the normal position. This can mean that there was nerve damage and should be examined by a physician immediately.

If the symptoms and/or pain are not that severe then the **Acute phase** may use the same procedures as outlined before including rest, icepacks, only pain-free movement, with anti-inflammatory medication such as *ibuprofen*. Progression is only appropriate when the back muscles can be activated isometrically without excessive pain. Again, excessive, consistent pain is a sign that one must consult a physician regarding the injury.

The *Rehab phase* will focus more on flexibility and strengthening of the back muscles. An effective stretch for all of the back muscles that are in direct attachment to the scapula is the Scapular Stretch. (Picture # 18.) One simply lies supine on the ground and laces his fingers behind his head. Then pull your elbows together which will create tension between the scapula muscles. ₄ Exercises that are effective include further action with the rope & pulley, and isotonic biceps curls and triceps extensions without weight will help too. Wall push-ups are effective in this phase and simply changing the distance one stands from the wall can easily change the intensity. For example, the further from the wall you are, the lower your hands will be, and the more weight that your exercise will bear.

Recovery phase can bear more resistance as with the T-Bar row that activates all the muscles in attachment to the scapula. Using the Butterfly, Elbow Abduction with more focused efforts on concentric movement, (muscle shortening), and this exercise can be an effective change in training of the Recovery phase (after confirming that the back is not injured). This allows one to change the *FIT* without having to use heavier dumbbells. One unique exercise that helps the strength training and endurance of your back rhomboid muscles is to use an arm cycling machine or seated rowing machine for several minutes.

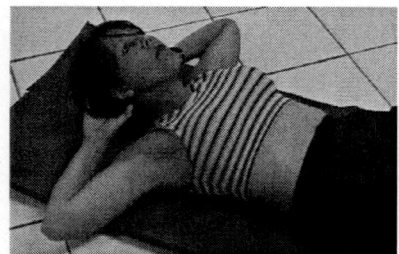
Pic #18, Scapular Stretch

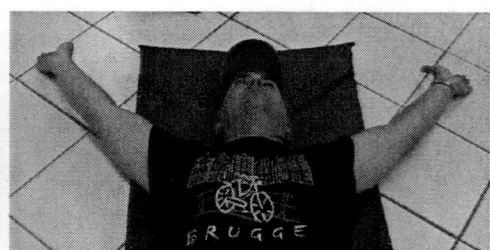
Pic #19, Shoulder stretch

In the final stage, strenuous exercises include Plyometric exercises with a medicine ball and an exercise called the

Glenohumoral extension. The Plyometric muscle activation refers to the process of extending the muscle to full length followed by a more powerful muscle contraction, (as done by Olympic high jumpers who drop to a low squat before jumping). One uses this technique by catching a medicine ball with the arms extended and then swinging the ball back to throw.

To perform the Glenohumoral extension exercise, one simply lies on his side (perhaps on the bed at first), and pushes the body up by extending the elbows. This is very strenuous and should only be used after one can accomplish all other exercises without pain. An effective, proactive exercise for scapular injury symptoms would be stretching and light muscle activation as with the rowing machine, and this will prevent future symptoms.

Scapular Injury Rehab summary
Acute phase: RICE
                Pain free movement
Rehab phase: Shoulder Blade stretch
                Wall Push-ups
                Isometric Biceps & triceps
Recovery: T-Bar rowing
                Elbow (Butterfly) Abduction
                Plyometric Medicine Ball
                Rowing Machine
                Glenohumoral extension

Shoulder Separation/Dislocation

Shoulder separation regularly occurs in contact sports and, or sports that require regular arm extension like gymnastics, and it should immediately require medical attention. But the following therapeutic exercises can be helpful in rehabilitating the shoulder so that dislocation may not happen again.

* It should be noted that if shoulder separation becomes frequent, the person might have a hyper-elasticity

problem that should be discussed with a physical medicine specialist.

After the medical care professionals have authorized starting rehabilitation, the person may begin the *Acute phase* training with efforts to regain the ROM. Again the broom handle may be used effectively to reach a 90-degree angle of abduction. Then move your arms through the normal coronal axis (parallel to the line from shoulder to shoulder).

The *Rehab phase* may begin again with the rope and pulley mechanism for resistance, neuromuscular control and gentle strength training. Exercises like this (and the simple knee raise for lower extremity injuries) are helpful because they are not too overt or strenuous, nor do they alter the body's normal movement patterns. Another protocol that will help the rehabilitation is to gently accomplish shoulder stretching. This is done by lying on the floor or bed and gently moving the hands along the side of the body until tension is felt. (Picture # 19.) Then one should hold that position for 20 seconds before moving back to a more comfortable position. These stretching sessions should be for 20 seconds with 4 to 6 repetitions of the stretch.

Strength training may begin with simple bar press, and at this time use only a broom handle so that the shoulder is not re-injured. Wall push-ups may also be used effectively to activate the appropriate muscles, as may the movement of a ball against a wall. (Picture #20.) This will also help retune the neuromuscular control.

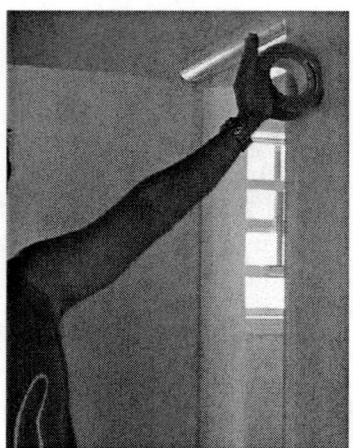

Pic #20, Ball on wall for NM control

60

During the *Recovery phase* one may also begin similar exercises as described for the *Recovery phase* of training for scapular injuries. Such advanced exercises include: T-Bar rowing, the Elbow (Butterfly) Abduction, Plyometric Medicine Ball, and using a Rowing Machine. However, the Glenohumoral extension should NOT be used as this can stress the connective tissue that holds the Glenohumoral head within the proper position.

Additional exercises in the *Recovery phase* of treating shoulder injuries includes lying elbow abduction/adduction with the lying Karate chop exercises, the Pectoral Fly exercise, the Latissimus dorsi pull down, and the military press. The Karate Chop Exercise begins by lying on your back, in bed and placing your wrists beside your head. Then "chop" your hands away from your head (abduction) to the surface of the bed. When the elbow is in that position, one should isometrically contract the muscles of the elbow, upper arm, and shoulder. (See picture #21, on the next page.)

The Pectoral Fly exercise can be done with either dumbbells or with a fly machine as shown in picture #22. This exercises the pectoral, chest muscle but uses the shoulder muscles as stabilizers, so this exercise is often used in proactive shoulder exercises (see chapter VII). The Military Press is performed by lifting a barbell above your head, while seated, and it also uses shoulder muscles to move the weight with upper pectoral muscles and the shoulder girdle also works as stabilizer muscles. The Latissimus Dorsi pull down (Lats Pull Down) uses the deltoids, and upper back rhomboid muscles, and this is an effective *Recovery* exercise or proactive exercise.

The military press is simply to press a barbell over your head while seated in an upright lifting chair. The primary action is to extend the arm while holding the barbell, and the movement is from your chest to full extension. Safety bars help control the descent of the bar in most apparatuses.

Scapular Injury Rehab, continued

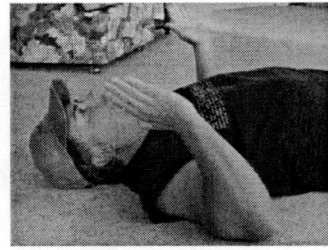 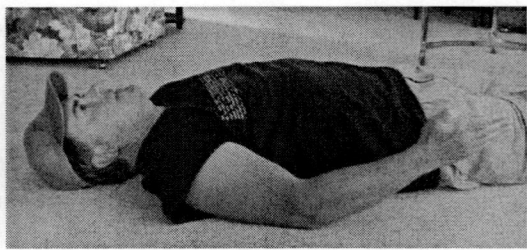

Pic #21 Karate Chop start   →   Finish

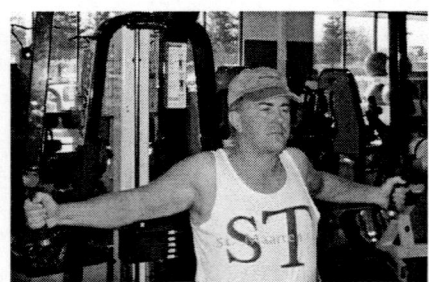 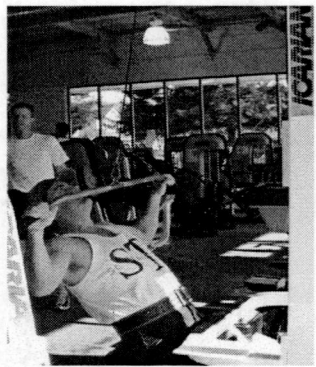

Pic #22 Pec Fly   **Pic #23** Lats Pull Down

ARM-ELBOW INJURIES

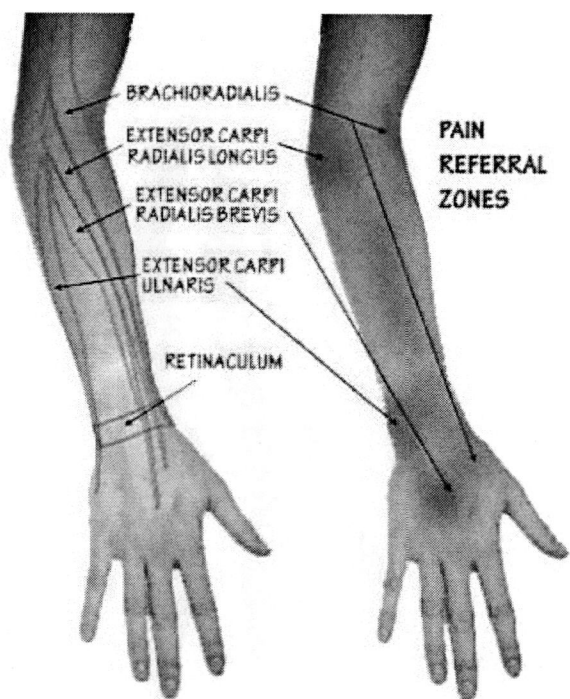

BRACHIORADIALIS

EXTENSOR CARPI
RADIALIS LONGUS

EXTENSOR CARPI
RADIALIS BREVIS

EXTENSOR CARPI
ULNARIS

RETINACULUM

PAIN
REFERRAL
ZONES

Figure #4, Lateral Epicondylitis, OrthoDoc, Massage

The elbow is as a joint with as complex musculature as the knee. See figure #1 and #2 for the upper torso muscles involved and notice the musculature at different depths from the skin's surface. Figure #4 shows the lateral extensor muscles that are symptomatic in Lateral Epicondylitis. The muscles must be activated too, because those muscles are also involved in the multiple-plane motions that the elbow moves through which include: flexion, extension, rotation, and circumduction.

These muscles from deep to superficial include: Coraco Brachialis, Brachialis, Brachioradialis, Bicipital Aponeurosis, Biceps Brachii, and the triceps Brachii. The exercises for strengthening the elbow after an injury may all seem similar but using different biomechanical components achieves the rehabilitation of different muscle groups.

Tennis Elbow (Lateral Epicondylitis)

This is the most common elbow injury that is caused by *Overuse* or unconditioned use of a repetitive movement of force such as swinging a tennis racket or a golf club, or swinging a baseball bat. [2,8,9,14,15]   Lateral Epicondylitis is diagnosed by pain and inflammation along the lateral extensor muscle mass near the tendon's insertion into bone. (See the dots along the brachioradialis and extensor carpi radialis muscles on figure #4.)

Common symptoms that are regularly associated with the *Overuse injuries* include the following: gradual onset of pain, pain directly over the outer elbow knob (lateral epicondyl), and increased pain upon rotation or impact. The most difficult portion of rehabilitation for lateral epicondylitis is to guarantee the rest and inactivity in the sport until rehabilitation training is complete in 3 weeks, and this is emotionally challenging for an avid sports enthusiast like one who plays tennis or golf. But, temporarily stopping participation in your sport of activity is an integral component of obtaining rehabilitation from this injury. That is part of the reason why this injury is common and almost chronic with avid tennis players, is because of their inability to stay off the tennis courts. This hampers their complete recovery, hence this is a reoccurring problem. As soon as the pain erupts, one must make the commitment for their recovery to stop playing tennis for 4 weeks while accomplishing rehabilitation, to avoid repeated onset of this injury. The **Acute phase** begins with *RICE*, and perhaps an anti inflammatory medication like *ibuprofen*. This should be continued for three days even though the pain will subside after a few hours.

After the third day of doing no more than pain free movement, then one may begin the complete training of the **Rehab phase.** Start each session with passive, static stretching. Once again that means to position the arm with your elbow on a horizontal surface (i.e. a table), and project the elbow far enough that the elbow and wrist are being stretched by gravity alone to full extension. (Picture # 24, next page.) Then you will need to stretch the extensor muscle, and this can be done with a "salute stretch" seen in picture #25. Both stretching should be done for 4 sets of 20 seconds. Then one may grab the back edge of the table with the knuckles up and use the structure for isometric muscle contraction.

In this isometric exercise, start the contractions from your fingertips and progress through your forearm muscles to the brachioradialis and biceps (biceps brachii). Hold the contraction for 20 seconds and do 4 sets of this exercise. Then begin with a multiple joint, multiple zoned movement with no significant weight. Do a biceps curl, beginning with a 12" ruler or empty coffee cup, and start the biceps contraction with your palms facing the anterior direction. Then curl the symptomatic elbow and flex the biceps while rotating the ruler until your thumb is pointed towards your face. (Picture #26.)

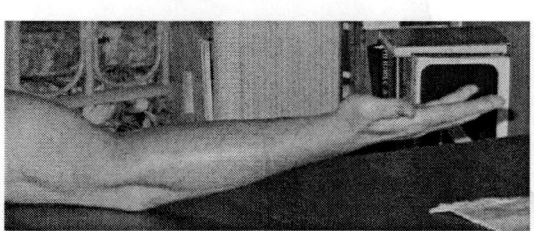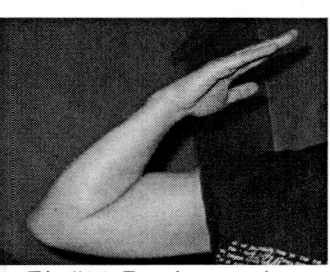

Pic #24, Passive, Static Elbow Extension Stretch   **Pic #25**, Passive, static Elbow Flexion stretch

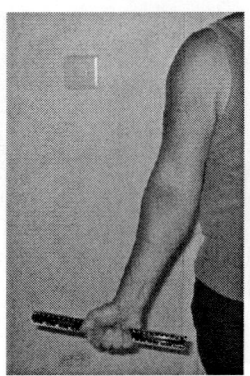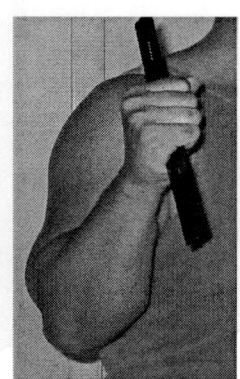

Pic #26 , Start biceps flex ➔ this Final position

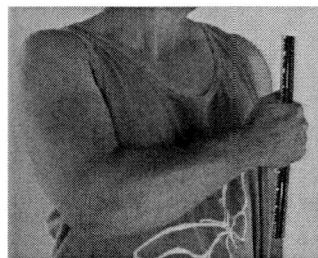

Start Biceps Flex   ➔   **Pic #27**, Alternate Bi-Flex Final position

65

After you are able to do Biceps flexion/rotation well without pain, then you can change the intensity by doing this exercise with a light dumbbell. For further variation, you can change the movement patter of this curl by moving your arm across your body so that the final position is with your extended thumb touching your opposite shoulder. (Picture # 27.) This will activate more muscles to regain the strength and symmetry for elbow flexion/extension. Finish your exercises with active stretching where you use the other hand to assist in stretching the elbow in flexion.

When you are ready for the **Recovery phase,** know that this work will seem tedious but it will benefit your performance and orthopedic health. A unique and very beneficial exercise is the *Hammer Rotation.* However, in this phase one should begin with a 12" inch ruler. One should begin with the forearm upon a table surface while holding the ruler in the medial side, and your palms facing the surface of the table. (Picture # 28, next page.) Then rotate the stick laterally until you feel tension. Then hold that position for 20 seconds, and you will have accomplished work for flexibility, neuromuscular control, and strength training of the Brachioradialis.

After successful training from day 4 to 10, then one can begin the **Recovery phase** of training for the tennis elbow or lateral Epicondylitis. Use a real Hammer in the previously described exercise and hold your forearm in mid air to avoid damaging your table with the hammerhead. As your strength increases and when there is no more pain, you may even try using extra resistance like wrapping an ankle weight around the hammerhead, but do this exercise with very slow movement.

Another effective exercise to be added to the stretching and hammer exercise is to move a medicine ball above your head in a lateral or coronal motion. This will strengthen a larger group of muscles that are the group used in different tennis strokes.

Tennis Elbow Rehab summary
Acute phase: FIRST 3 DAYS
(RICE)
Passive, Static Stretching

Rehab phase: DAY 3 to SECOND WEEK
Isometrics
Biceps flexion/rotation
Recovery: WEEKS 3 to 6
Stick rotation
Lateral Hammer rotation
Overhead Medicine Ball

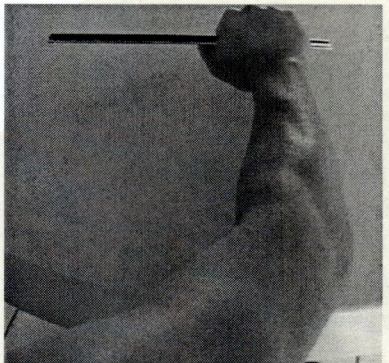 →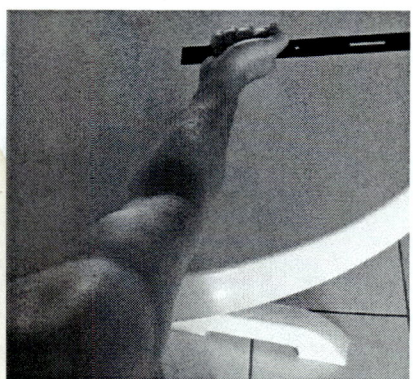

Pic #28, Lateral Hammer rotation → Final position

Golfer's Elbow Syndrome

Again the most difficult part of rehabilitating dedicated golfers of this disorder is the fact that they must stay off the links for more than two weeks. The exercises are very similar to the simple lateral Epicondylitis previously described, but there are significant biomechanical differences.

Begin the ***Acute phase*** with RICE and just passive static stretching for the elbow, combined with active stretching of the shoulder. Wear the bandage for three days, and apply ice every evening. Then one may start the ***Rehab phase*** with the similar isometric contractions against a table as for tennis elbow. Then adapt the lateral stick rotation movement for golfer's elbow syndrome by starting with your stick in an opposite position. Start with the stick to the lateral side so that the concentric movement is towards the medial side. (Picture # 29.) This

67

effects a different cadence of muscular contractions that
simulates part of the golf swing.

As you begin the ***Recovery phase*** you will need to work
your wrists in three separate, distinct motions while flexing and
extending your elbow. First, begin with a Hammer curl. Use a
ruler or light dumbbell while seated and start with your arm
extended and the dumbbell heads front to back. Then flex your
biceps and bring the dumbbell to an elevated position, just as
one would bring up a hammer. In a separate exercise for
different muscle isolation, complete a dumbbell extension across
your chest (heads high and low). Start with the dumbbell at
your chest and then extend your arm completely. (Picture # 30.)

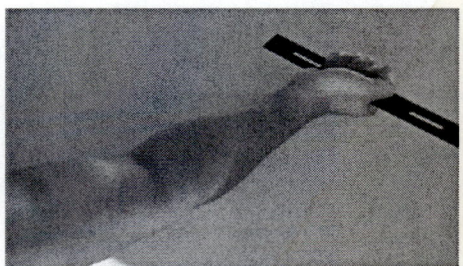 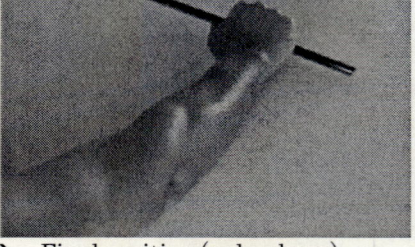

Pic #29 - **Golf's** Hammer rotation start ➔ Final position (palm down)

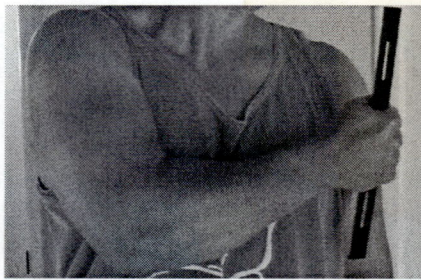 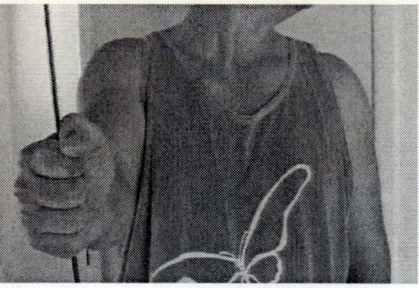

Pic # 30 Dumbbell Extension start ➔ Full Extension

The third movement for this exercise regime is to lean
over and rotate the dumbbell in a circular pattern,
(circumduction). This will effectively strengthen the muscles
used for rotation in your golf swing. Another exercise that will
be useful is to hold your hands on opposite sides of the medicine
ball and simulate a golf swing. First use the regular swing as

the concentric position of the exercise, and then reverse it by beginning with the ball high as forcing it down in an opposite swinging movement.

A final exercise for strengthening the forearm muscles would be to "Wind Up" a rope with weight on it. Begin with a 12-inch broomstick, and tie one end of the stick to the rope and one end to a gallon carton, that is half full of water (a half gallon of water weighs 4lbs). Simply wind and unwind the 36 inches of rope, slowly in two different wrist positions (one palm up and one with palm down). In one winding position have your elbows tucked beside you and in the other position have you arms totally extended for the action. When ready to increase the intensity, increase the resistance to a full gallon of water (which equals 8lbs).

Golfer's syndrome, Rehab summary

Acute phase: RICE
          Passive, Static Stretching
Rehab phase: Isometrics
          Opposite stick and Hammer
Recovery: Wrist Exercises (3 planes)
          Medicine Ball swing
          Wind Up weight

Pitcher's Elbow

This disorder again has components of Lateral Epicondylitis, but also has a unique pathology that includes the mechanical function of the shoulder plus elbow plus the wrist movement. [6] The protocols will be similar but this disorder uses different exercises and more stretching of the wrist muscles.

The *Acute phase* is key on the use of ice for inflammation but is less dependant on restricting compression as the maximum ROM is important to maintain. For this syndrome only use the compression bandages while sleeping, (unless the pain is so severe that you must use it during the day). Again use the gentle flexing techniques, but also use the yardstick or golf club to move the arm through the fullest range of motion possible without pain.

When starting the **Rehab phase** one must utilize the stretching techniques for the shoulder (see rotator cuff section), the active elbow stretching, and at least two wrist stretching techniques. The first wrist stretching technique is for the wrist flexors. 6 Stand over a table and place your hands in alignment side-by-side upon the table. Then lean your body beyond your hands, which will achieve the tension for stretching. Hold this position for 20 seconds and accomplish 4 sets, twice per day.

Now lift your hands with your palm facing your face, and use your other hand to actively stretch the wrist in flexion. These two stretching protocols stretch both the muscles for extension and flexion, and the following strength training will also work the flexor and extensor muscles.

An elastic band is the most efficient for isolated wrist strength training. Simply stand on one end and loop the other end of the elastic cord around your wrist. Do four sets of flexion contractions and 4 sets of extension contractions. Then continue with the exercises for lateral Epicondylitis previously described, including: Hammer rotation, Biceps Flexion rotation, and use a stick to simulate the movement of "Joystick flight controls."

Recovery phase, begin the "joystick" exercise by putting one end of a broomstick between your feet. Simply grab the top of the handle with the injured arm and move the stick in to each number on an imaginary clock. Go from center to 1 o'clock, to center, to 2 o'clock, etc. For an advanced exercise with this movement, do the motions while isometrically contracting the resistant (antagonistic) muscles. This will help regain the symmetry for activation during throwing.

The phase will add an exercise of holding a single dumbbell with both hands, above your head, (one hand on each dumbbell head). This will activate the shoulder muscles used for stability right before release of the baseball. Another exercise that uniquely activates many of the forearm and humoral muscles is the Butterfly Dumbbell Abduction exercise, described on pages 57 and 58.

Additional Exercises for the arm and elbow injuries would include the towel twist and elbow extensions. The towel twist begins with one standing and holding out the towel with your forearms extended. Then twist the towel to your maximum ability in one direction, and follow that with unwinding and winding in the opposite direction. Elbow extension exercises can

70

be done seated with the wrist moving outward as shown in picture #30, or the motion may be lateral, with movement of the wrist and stick along the lateral axis.

Pitcher's Elbow Rehab summary

Acute phase:	FIRST 3 DAYS
	RICE (compression pm)
	Passive, Static Stretching
Rehab phase:	DAYS 4 TO 14
	2 Wrist stretches
	Wrist resistance exercises
	Hammer rotation
Recovery:	WEEKS 3 TO 6
	Dumbbell balance overhead
	Joystick simulation with
	Isometric contractions
	Towel twisting

WRIST/HAND

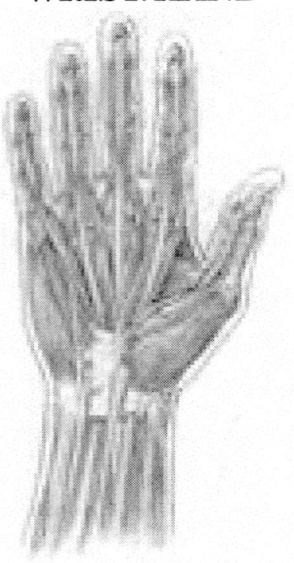

Figure 5, Wrist/Hand musculature

Wrist Tendonitis

This condition frequently occurs after repeatedly hitting or punching, (as done by a boxer), by repeatedly throwing a ball or this may occur from a traumatic impact injury.

The *Acute* phase of treatment begins with *RICE* and passive, static stretching. Try only to stretch in one direction at a time because rotating the wrist around can cause more damage to the connective tissue, (the ligaments and tendons of the wrist).

In the *Rehab phase,* regaining ROM is key, but one must work gently because there is not great direct blood supply to the wrist bones, which makes the recovery and healing time longer. An effective excise is the rope and pulley, which activates both the key flexor and extensor muscles of the hand and wrist. A unique exercise is the Power grip, (Picture # 31). This is done by grasping a mesh of elastic cables, (which also activates the finger flexors to help strengthen the tendons), then after closing your fist, rotate it 45 degrees. This will help regain ROM, strength, neuro-motor control and strength simultaneously.

Upon starting the *Recovery phase* isometric and fixed resistance exercises are very beneficial. Using fixed resistance such as pushing against a wall, or working to extend your hand against a wall are more effective than the few resistance exercises that are rarely available. Working with rope grips and pulley mechanisms also help train the muscles attached to the symptomatic tendons for a more complete recovery.

<u>Wrist Tendonitis Rehab summary</u>
Acute phase: RICE
               Passive, Static stretch
Rehab phase: Rope Pulley
               Flexibility all planes
               Power grip
Recovery: Isometrics
               Fixed resistance exercise
               Grip & Pull

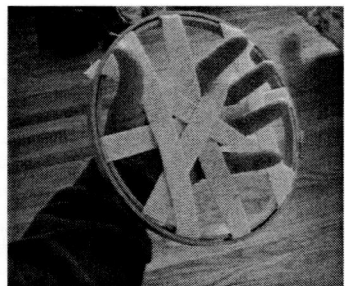

Pic# 31 Power Grip   →

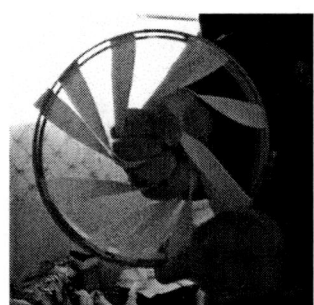

Contraction and Twist

<u>Skier's Wrist (Ulnar collateral ligament damage)</u>

This is often called the Skier's wrist, and it is seen by the symptom of having pain from wrist to thumb. The *Acute phase* begins with *RICE,* but one must be careful not to have the compression garment too tight. Reducing the already poor blood flow can be catastrophic. Often immobilization of the thumb and medical care are required for this injury. However, the following protocols are effective in rehabilitating the wrist after

73

immobilization has been stopped and your medical professional authorizes the rehab training.

Begin the *Rehab phase* by simply holding a tennis ball. Then move the tennis ball over a table surface with your palm in constant contact with the ball. This will regain neuromuscular control while increasing the blood flow. After the pain has subsided in this phase, one may combine this ball-rolling with squeezing of the ball.

The *Recovery phase* can also effectively use the Power grip device exercise. This can also be combined with rotation of the wrist to strengthen the muscles and tendons to avoid repeated injury of this area. Now one can roll a volleyball against a wall. This will train the wrist extensors and the collateral ligaments of the wrist. (See picture # 20.) The rolling can also include isometric or fixed resistance exercises as well. An additional exercise in this phase would be the towel twist as described in the elbow injury section, but this can be more effectively done with the towel upright, with one hand above the other.

The recovery of this injury can be lengthy, but long recovery would be better than having an injury that continually reoccurs.

Skier's Wrist Rehab summary

Acute phase:	DAY 1 TO 3
	Medical Treatment
	RICE
	Immobilize thumb
Rehab phase:	DAYS 4 TO 14
	Tennis ball rolling
	Rolling + squeeze
Recovery:	WEEKS 3 to 6
	Power grip
	Volleyball on wall
	Power grip + rotation
	or Upright Towel Twists

Chapter IV (L)
Exercise Therapies, Lower Extremities

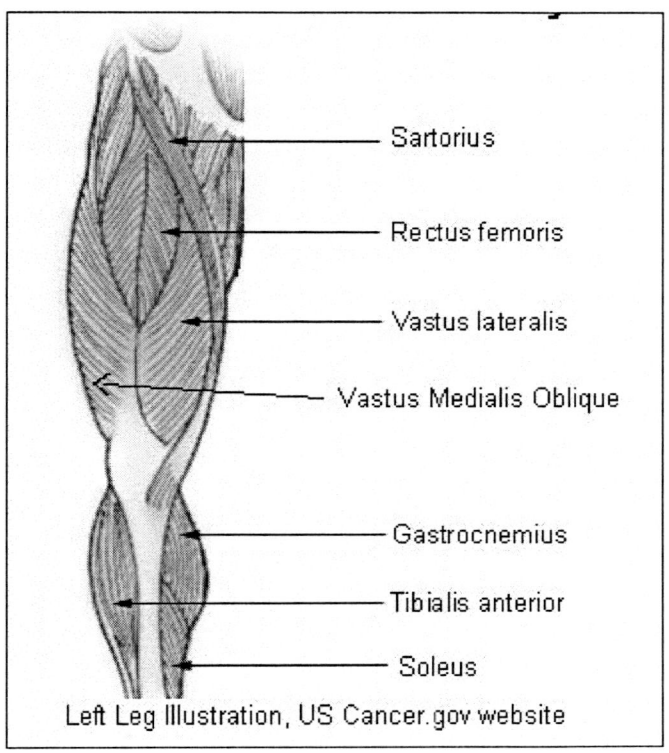

Left Leg Illustration, US Cancer.gov website

Figure #6, Lower Extremity musculature

Rehabilitation of Lower Extremities

This chapter will reveal exercises therapy programs that have been designed to treat the common, orthopedic injuries of your lower extremities. Rehabilitation of the lower extremities must also include thought on your complete lifestyle and other activities because normal mobility also requires strength and endurance of your injured extremities. The timing of when you train and when you do your normal walking may require forethought after you stop using crutches or other devices. In my rehab therapy, I noticed that accomplishing my rehab training first thing in the morning was more productive and left me feeling better for the rest of the day. When I was progressing in how much weight I could bear on the ankle (that had recently been fused), I noticed that if I did more weight bearing in the morning and then used the crutches more fully in the afternoon, it allowed me to go with less pain medication. The neural blocker pain medication also inhibits bone deposition, so taking less pain meds helped my progression excel.

Examine your normal schedule of walking to work, school, grocery stores, park walking, etc., and plan on the times when you will be overly fatigued after training so that your rehab efforts enhance your lifestyle rather than detract from it.

Exercise Therapies

This section will address the lower extremities of the body and include therapeutic protocols for treating common injuries in those areas, and it will describe the majority of therapeutic protocols for treating the injury with the primary components for acquiring complete rehabilitation training. Those components to be acquired are: Range of Motion (ROM), Neuromuscular activation, Flexibility training, Strength training, and Proactive exercises. Each injury treatments' description will include a summary of the phases and exercises benefiting that region and injury.

Hip, Thigh Injuries

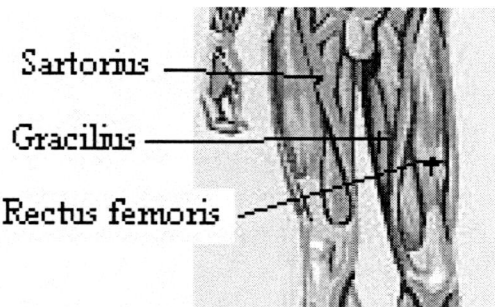

Sartorius

Gracilius

Rectus femoris

Figure #7, Gracilius illustration

Gracilius "Groin" Strain

This is a common injury that occurs as a painful crisis following running or jumping. The groin muscle seen in Figure #7 is not the primary muscle used in the movements of running and/or jumping but, after one's quadriceps are fatigued, the body then recruits the groin muscle (Gracilius) which is easily strained and/or torn. The symptoms when the fibers have been torn include sharp, stabbing pains and the inability to move the leg inward, (followed by bruising in a day or two). Less acute injuries may show high levels of soreness hours after injuring the muscle and pain when retracting the leg to the rear.

Caution should be taken to ensure that these symptoms of groin pain are not from other causes, which could be: Stress fractures of the thigh bone (femur), Tumors, and Hernias. If there are other significant symptoms (other than the ones listed above), you should definitely have a health care professional investigate your injury.

After you have determined that the condition is only a groin strain, then the *Acute phase's* initial treatment would be *RICE.* The compression bandage should not be too tight, and can be applied to the upper thigh(s). Lying on one's back, with slight elevation of the pelvic area and both legs will help to reduce the pain, inflammation, and swelling. Ice packs on the injured area will also be effective. Movement should be gentle and not assisted in any way.

In the *Rehab phase,* one can begin working with different, effective stretches if the injury was not acute. Moving to the ground for said stretching may yield pain and difficulty in arising, so begin the stretching while on an elevated surface such as a treatment table or bed. The first will be the regular "Groin stretch" is also described as the Pelvic Adductor stretch, and the alternate hand placement in this stretch affects the primary muscle fibers that are stretched. Putting one hands on top of the feet while bending forward will stretch the deeper, higher (more proximal) muscles than the traditional position with one's hands on the ankles and elbows pushing down on the knees. (Picture #32) Use both techniques for a more completely stretched groin muscle (Gracilius).

A unique stretch that will be used is the Supine Piriformis stretch. To do this, lay on your back, and bend the knee of one leg to 90 degrees. Then allow that leg to fold over the other leg to accomplish the tension for this stretch, (Picture #33.) This stretched the Gracilius and supportive tissue with the deeper muscle the Pirisiformis that lies deeper in the region of the Gracilius origin. Another flexibility exercise will be the Supine Knee Tuck, (Picture #34) To accomplish this stretch, simply lie on your back and pull both knees to your chest.

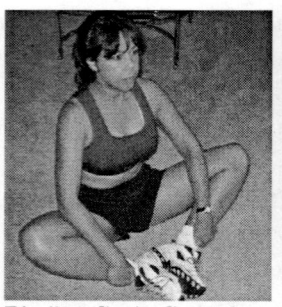 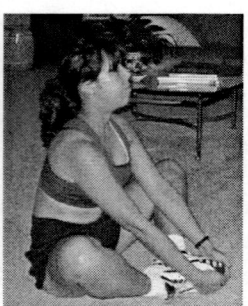

Pic #32 Groin Stretch   Alternate Hand placement

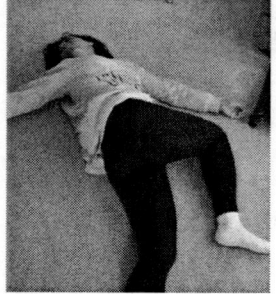

Pic #33 Piriformis stretch

Once the flexibility training has concluded, then one can begin with some unique strengthening exercises that also enhance neuromuscular training. The first such exercise is simply to compress a pillow between one's knees. As the rehab progresses one can change the *FIT* in three ways: *Frequency can be* changed by doing this exercise twice daily, and for changing the *Intensity,* you can add another pillow for greater resistance. The duration that you train can be longer, thus changing the *Time* spent exercising.

Simply standing on one leg is effective for strengthening the Gracilius, and it is also effective for the neuromuscular control. Stand on each individual leg, even if the injury seems to be more severe on one side. Another effective exercise that uses the Gracilius as a stabilizer is to lie on the side and lift (abduct) the top leg with an ankle weight. Perform this exercise on both legs and it will be effective for this phase of treatment.

In the **Recovery phase** one can benefit greatly from deep squats, using a Smith (squat) Machine ® for safety and stability. Begin with no weight and only holding onto the bar for support. Do less than 6 such squats to the full depth (the knee joint angle of 90°), and after a few days, you can add more free squats and, you can slightly change the foot position width or change the depth of your free squats. Holding onto the support bar while squatting with zero weight will keep from re-injuring the Gracilius, because that keeps the Gracilius from being activated preferentially. After doing these free squats for a week, you can increase the intensity by now squatting with the bar on a Smith Machine, but additional weight should not be added until beginning the 3rd week of the Rehab phase. When the weight is added, remember the saying, "Better too light than too heavy."

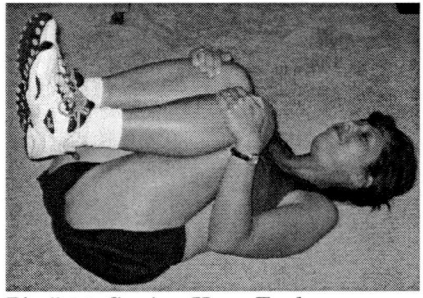
Pic # 34, Supine Knee Tuck

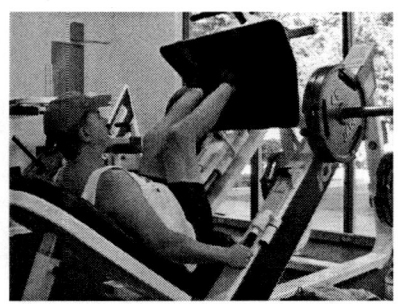
Pic #35 Incline Leg Extension Sled

Other exercises for the recovery phase may include using a resistance band for leg adduction and ski machines are effective because they allow smooth abduction of the legs, which should reduce the repeat onset of this injury. Machines such as an incline leg extension sled will allow the addition of free weight, and this is also effective for isolating the Gracilius and Sartorius, (Picture #35). For isolation, the foot placement must be in natural alignment but just more than shoulder-width apart. For final neuromuscular control training, one can stand on a wobble board (see picture #46 on page 103), which would be effective unless the person has had ankle problems.

Even during the Recovery phase, one should begin with sets of two stretching protocols, then train for strengthening and increased neuromuscular control, and then finish with two different sets of stretching protocols.

Gracilius "Groin" Strain Rehab Summary

Acute Phase:	FIRST 3 DAYS
	R.I.C.E.
	Passive, static stretching
	Light massage
Rehab Phase:	DAYS 3 TO 14
	Four Stretching Protocols
	Pillow Compression
	Standing One leg
	Ankle weight Abduction
Recovery:	WEEKS 3 TO 6
	Flexibility x 2
	Free squat (No weight)
	Hip Flexor band
	Incline Leg extension sled
	Flexibility x 2

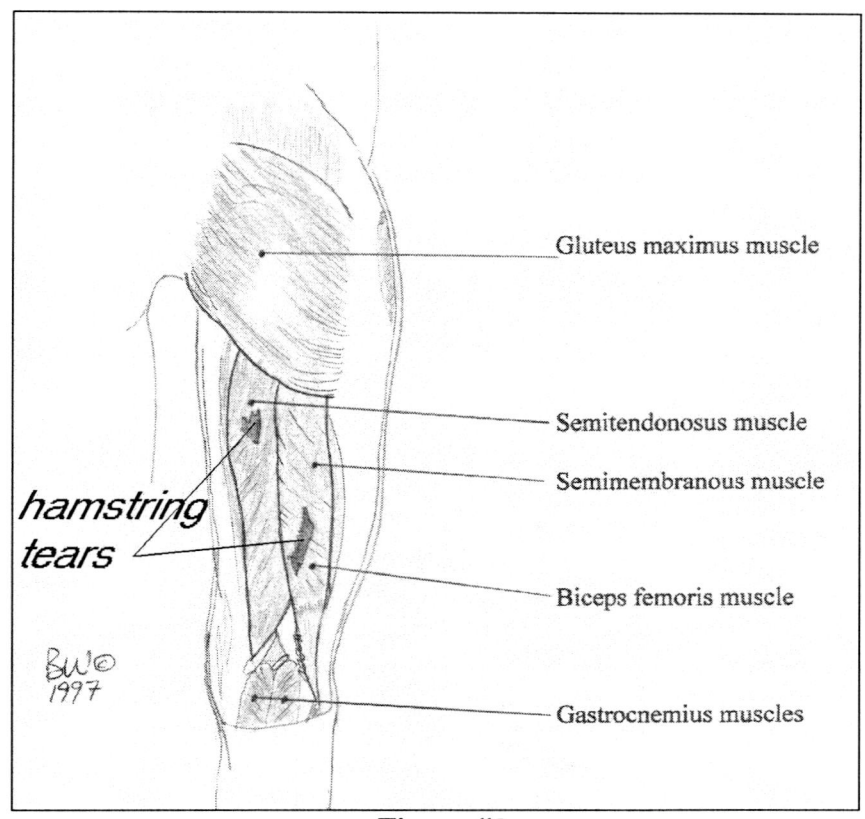

Gluteus maximus muscle

Semitendonosus muscle

Semimembranous muscle

hamstring tears

Biceps femoris muscle

BW©
1997

Gastrocnemius muscles

Figure #8

Hamstring Pull or Tear

A Hamstring pull or tear is an injury that affects athletes who participate in fast-start sports, (like in American Football or Soccer). When one says that they have a "Hamstring tear or pull," that is an injury to the area of the ischial tuberosity (lower pelvis bone), or the "hamstrings" (biceps femoris and semitendinosis muscles). Such a "Pull" is less severe than a "Tear," because a tear includes rupture of musculature, as seen in the illustration above. A tear will usually show bruising in a few days, from the concurrent rupture of arterioles.

The *Acute phase* treatment is focused on *RICE.* The immediate Rest, Ice, Compression (wrap the elastic bandage around the thigh), and Elevation are integral factors for reducing pain, inflammation, swelling, pain. Pain-free stretching can be done in this phase, and the hamstring stretch described earlier, is also very effective. Also one may begin slow, isometric contractions, knee flexion, and the straight leg raise exercise (if the injury is less severe). (See picture #39, page 86.) Towards the latter days of this phase, one can even begin Supine marching, where one simply accomplishes the leg movements of marching while lying supine on the bed.

In the *Rehab phase* one may begin with assisted stretching of the hamstrings by using a towel on the ball of the foot. Walking slowly with crutches or a walker-device, with very little weight upon the injured leg is very effective for neuromuscular control and for strengthening the muscles for stabilization, which include the hamstrings, gracilius, and sartorius. In the second week of this phase, one might begin doing this while the feet are on a balance platform or wobble board with the crutches which help supply stability.

After the isometric contractions can be completed with little pain, then light resistance such as elastic cables may be used, as long as the pain is low and the pain does not have peaks during the exercise. Since weight bearing is painful with this injury, one may find great success with aquatic therapy. One may simply get into a swimming pool and slowly do the freestyle kick, while holding onto the wall.

During the *Recovery phase* a new exercise may be used which is the Isokinetic machine for knee flexion and extension. This piece of equipment relies on the cadence of movement with resistance and it requires a specific force production throughout the movements. The equipment is regularly available in a sports medicine clinic or physical therapy clinic. Another exercise that keeps one from bearing the full body weight is the stationary bicycle. The Interval or Random resistance programs are the best to use, preferably on a LifeFitness Lifecycle ®. This is effective because the contractions allow the muscles to exert high force, but then also allowing recuperative time to rest from high-force production.

Again the flexibility training should be used before and after all strength training, and changes in the order of exercises done will be helpful as well. Effective isotonic exercises for the hamstrings also includes the hamstring curl or knee flexion that was performed isometrically. Isotonic means that one does the exercise with resistance as seen here, on picture #36.

Hamstring pull or tear, Rehab Summary

Acute phase: RICE
　　　　　　ROM flexibility
　　　　　　Pain Free Ham stretching
　　　　　　Supine marching
Rehab phase: Standing on crutches
　　　　　　Isometric contractions
　　　　　　Aquatic therapy
Recovery: 　Isokinetic Machine
　　　　　　Lifecycle
　　　　　　Hamstring curls

Some additional exercises for hip & thigh injuries include a Leg Slide. Lie supine (with the back on a the floor or bed), and extend your legs, followed by flexing your legs (abduction & adduction). This is beneficial for the hip flexors and extensors. Then one might do the knee/ankle abduction, where one sits on a bench or chair, holds the knees together and then separates the ankles. Another advanced, *recovery phase* exercise is to do the Standing Knee to Chest exercises, where you simply stand and elevate your knees as high as possible. (Picture #37.)

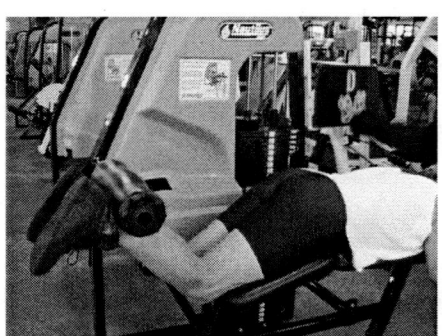

Pic #36 Prone Hamstring Curl

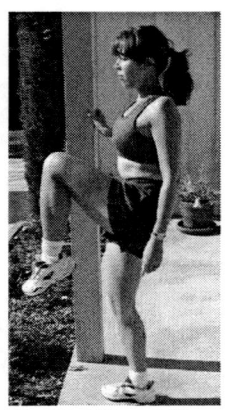

Pic #37 Stand Knee to Chest

KNEE INJURIES

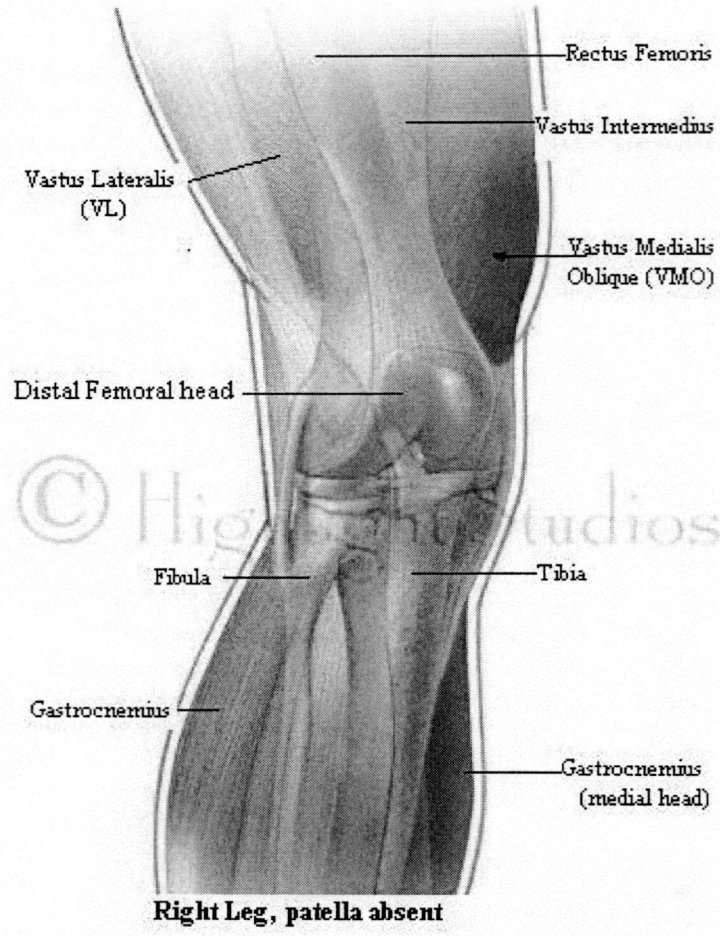

Rectus Femoris

Vastus Intermedius

Vastus Lateralis
(VL)

Vastus Medialis
Oblique (VMO)

Distal Femoral head

Fibula

Tibia

Gastrocnemius

Gastrocnemius
(medial head)

Right Leg, patella absent
Figure #9, Knee Musculature

A key component of most all knee injuries is atrophy of the inner knee muscle, the Vastus Medialis Oblique muscle, (or VMO as seen in this illustration). Atrophy is a decrease in the muscles' diameter, which coincides with the muscles' decreased strength. This is often either the cause, effect, or side effect from a knee injury. [1,2,3,6,9,11,12, 14]

Knee Contusion Injury

This is impact upon the knee (particularly from the lateral side), which results in bleeding beneath the skin (subcutaneous), and often results in VMO muscle atrophy. The Symptoms frequently include immediate pain after the collision, swelling and stiffness, and bruising after a few days, (bleeding below the skin surface is symptom of the contusion injury).

Beginning the *Acute phase* treatment with *RICE* is imperative and *RICE* is an almost mandatory treatment for knee injuries. [1,3,8,12] Begin with Rest from excess movement and rest from bearing your weight, obtain light Compression bandage such as an Ace® elastic bandage, and apply Ice packs as the knee is resting in the Elevated position. This should be done for the first 24-48 hours or until the pain has abated.

If the injury makes walking painful, crutches will be required (crutches can be found at most pharmacies). It is important to avoid being "too tough" with the knee injury because inadequately treated knee injuries are a leading cause to further, more severe knee disorders and injuries. [1,2,3,12] In the first three days one should only attempt light, knee flexion & stretching, but do that many times each day.

To accomplish light stretching, lie flat on your back with your femur (upper leg bone) in a vertical position. Then simply allows gravity to achieve the greatest flexion of the bent knee, before experiencing pain (See the Gentle Quad stretch Pic #38, next page.) Measuring and recording the maximum flexion is also important to establish clinical progression. The average, maximal knee flexion in a health adult is to approximately 30° - 40° of flexion. (This measurement is the small angle between the femur and tibia while the knee is flexed, and in comparison, the fully extended position is 180 degrees.)

Treatment in the *Rehab phase* is to allow increased movement without forcing the knee to bear body weight. This phase will also be focused on "Open-chain" exercises, which are exercises that keep the foot from bearing weight in contact with a fixed surface. The key beginning exercise for knee therapy is the straight leg raise, (SLR). The SLR should be done with as much extension as one can bear. So the order of the exercise is to lift the heel of one's foot while simultaneously extending the leg and contracting all muscles. (Picture #39)

The intensity of the SLR exercise can be changed by simply increasing the force of contraction while lifting, and later the leg can be raised with weight and/or isometric speed of contraction. The extension/flexion of the knee joint is so important that frequently after Anterior Cruciate Ligament (ACL) surgical repair, the patient will be placed in a knee flexion/extension machine for constant movement before even "waking-up" from the anesthetics.

The next exercise that will be used throughout treatment for all the knee injuries is riding a stationary cycle. The first goal will be to complete a full revolution of the pedals. If it is too painful to complete a full revolution/cycle, then simply "rock" or swing your pedal position from one side to the other side before reaching the painful zones. (Picture #40) This exercise will easily allow one to increase muscle activation, increase the flood flow, and this will begin to strengthen the injured muscles without bearing full weight.

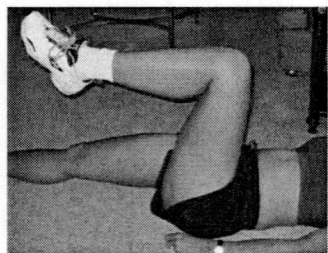

Pic #38 Gentle Quad Stretch

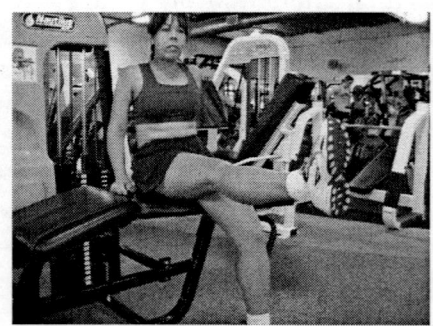

Pic #39 Straight Leg raise

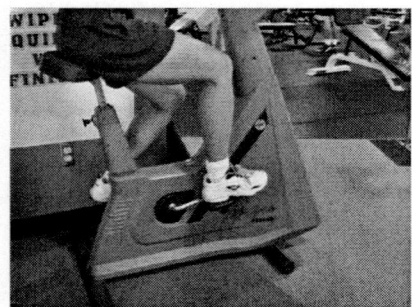

Pic #40 Pedal Rock:
      Rock pedal to the rear

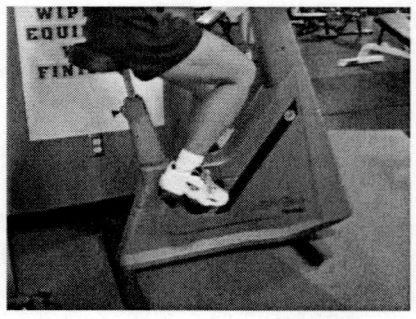

→   This position (before pain hits)

Once one can complete the revolution and comfortably cycle for 5 minutes, then one must begin the Open Stance Cycling Protocol, (OSCP), designed by the author for substantially increased VMO activation to counteract the VMO atrophy with an open-chained exercise. The protocol simply starts with a unique foot position on the pedal, and that yields a biomechanical change. The foot alignment is forward with the calcaneus bone (Heel) above the middle of the pedal (pedal axis) and the foot in an open or "Plie" position of 45 degrees more open than the direction of the cycle.

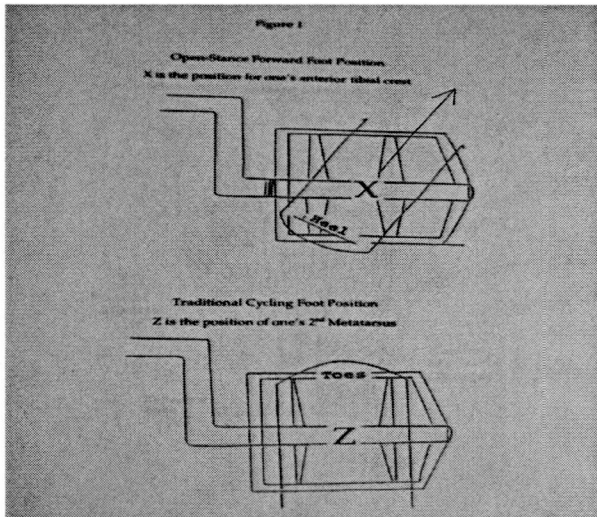

Figure #10, OSCP foot position, BW 1997

This biomechanical change has been shown to achieve preferential VMO activation in both healthy and symptomatic subjects. [3,6]

Begin cycling in five-minute segments, and when comfortable, increase the time by additional 5-minute intervals, every week. Changing the *FIT* should only be done once per week. Also, continue using the SLR but add ankle weights or elastic band upon the ankle for light resistance to extension, if you are pain free in this exercise.

Once you can walk comfortably and your knee flexion is within ten degrees of normal flexion, (test your other knee for comparison), then one can begin the *Recovery phase.* During the recovery phase you can work more vigorous exercises, including closed-chained exercises. Closed-chained exercises are exercises where one has a fixed foot position while performing an exercise, i.e. squatting a barbell with weights. For an example of closed-chained vs. open-chained exercises, compare the barbell squat with the SLR. The SLR is an open chained exercise because the foot is free from weight bearing. (See picture #39). In this recovery phase one must continue SLR and the OSCP exercises, and a *FIT* change with the OSCP is easily accomplished by riding with a "random" program of resistance, as seen with the Lifecycle.®

Further exercises for the *recovery phase* include squatting, but this is best done with a "Smith machine" squat rack. This apparatus controls the movement so that there is only one axis of motion, up and down. This achieves full muscle activation without risking further injury. Another effective exercise for later motor unit control, is side walking. This activates different support/position muscles and it helps the walking pattern (gait), to become smoother. Further exercises can include the leg extension weight machine, the leg extension/upright weight-sled, and the isokinetic knee flexion/extension machine.

The key point to remember is safety first, and a slow, thorough rehabilitative period will achieve a more thorough, longer lasting recovery. The OSCP has been described as an effective, proactive exercise to symptomatic conditions, such as "stadium seating" which is symptomatic with VMO atrophy and most knee injuries. [1,2,3,6,9]

Knee Contusion Injury

Acute Phase: RICE is imperative
 Use CRUTCHES if needed
 Passive Knee Flex/stretching

Rehab Phase: Quadriceps stretching
 Straight leg Raise
 Pedal Rock
 Open Stance Cycling

Recovery: SLR & OSCP
 Smith Squats
 Side Walking

88

Patellofemoral pain syndrome

Patellofemoral pain syndrome (PFPS) is most often associated with chronic knee-pain conditions, however, it often may be the underlying cause of repeated knee injuries, due to a muscular asymmetry. The primary symptom of this condition is having pain while ascending or descending stairs or pain from long durations of being seated, and that is often called pain from "stadium seating." [3,6,9,12] Other symptoms include pain in front of the kneecap (patella), a crunching or crackling sensation when bending the knee, and people with PFPS often complain that their knee "gives out." Often patients with PFPS suffer patellar subluxation, which is pain from the lateral glide of the patella.

The *Acute phase* can be any time of re-injuring the knee or any time that the symptoms of PFPS are acute and/or intense. As with most knee injuries *RICE* will be important to avoid further injury and increased symptoms. During this time one may also perform passive knee extension/flexion and passive stretching exercises. Since this may not be the first time of knee pain and injury, one may also benefit from cycling at a slow pace (1 revolution should take 2 seconds or 30 rmp), and no resistance should be used at this time.

During the *Rehab phase* one will benefit greatly from preferential VMO training that can be accomplished by using the Open Stance Cycling Protocol (OSCP) and the weighted SLR. The OSCP can increase the VMO activation by keeping the foot in the *plie* alignment as done on OSCP. Continue the flexibility training and SLR with increased intensity.

The *Recovery phase* will include increasing the *FIT* of the OSCP. This will continue to challenge the VMO, which will increase the muscle activation, strength and size. During this phase, frequently do isometric flexion of the quadriceps, and see figure #9 for clear pictures of the VMO and VL that show the biomechanical muscle alignment.

Individual leg training is effective during the recovery phase, and it will keep the weaker knee from relying upon the stronger, which is common in chronic conditions of muscular asymmetry. [9,11,12] Use a knee extension machine (Picture #42) that has rollers to allow for free movement through the exercise, and do single repetitions. Begin with the lightest weight and it may be required to start with zero weight. Focus on the slower concentric (muscle shortening) contraction motion during the quadriceps contraction. This will yield greater recruitment of the muscle for greater strength training.

Smith Squats are still effective here and, try to accomplish the squats to varying depths. On some days, try heavier weight and limit the flexion to only a 15-degree depth of knee flexion. This will train the distal quadriceps. Then try the smith machine with no weight but with as full and deep of a squat as can be obtained. This will recruit the more proximal femoral muscles such as rectus femoris, Sartorius, and Gracilius. Be careful though that you do not injure these muscles that are so rarely activated preferentially.

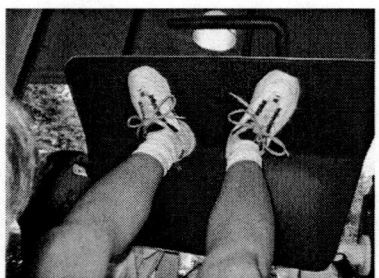
Pic #41 Plie footing on Sled

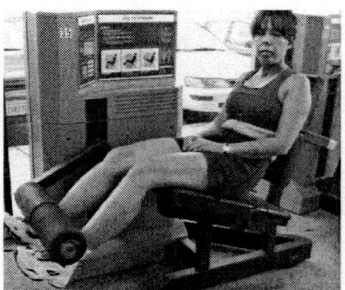
Pic #42 Knee Extension machine

Patellofemoral pain syndrome, Summary

Acute Phase: RICE
Passive Knee Flex/stretching
Cycle for ROM, no resistance

Rehab Phase: Straight leg Raise
Open Stance Cycling protocol
Weighted SLR

Recovery: OSCP
Resistance individual knee
extensions
Smith Squats, varying squat
depth
Incline Leg extension sled

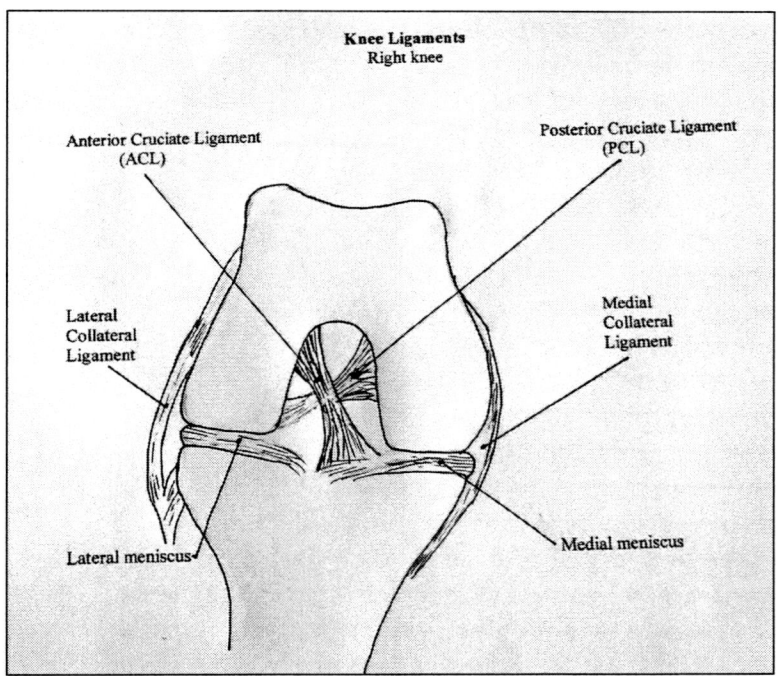

Knee Ligaments
Right knee

Anterior Cruciate Ligament
(ACL)

Posterior Cruciate Ligament
(PCL)

Lateral
Collateral
Ligament

Medial
Collateral
Ligament

Lateral meniscus

Medial meniscus

Figure #11, Ligaments of Flexed Knee

Knee Ligament Sprains or Tears

Frequently ligament sprains are the result of a contusion injury or from an incident where the knee joint may have become severely hyper-extended. A tear is an injury that should be medically treated, but both a sprain and tear (after surgical repair) will benefit from these rehab phases. The Anterior Cruciate Ligament (ACL), the Lateral Cruciate Ligaments (LCL), and the Medial Cruciate Ligaments (MCL), are frequently injured, and the symptoms of ligament tears include immediate pain after the injury, swelling, stiffness. With an ACL tear, one often hears or feels a "Pop" sound.

The *Acute phase* must begin with *RICE,* and as soon as the pain has abated, you may begin gentle flexion/extension movement. To do this, simply place your ankle on a towel, above a firm surface such as a board, and slowly pull the towel towards you by flexing your knee. This will accomplish the gentle knee flexion, and for extension, simply let gravity and your relaxation return the knee to an extended position.

During the **Rehab phase** a simple Straight Leg raise movement may be beneficial. One should still continue the flexion & extension exercises, and if possible gently working on a stationary bicycle will help too. This cycling should only try to gain full range of motion through the bicycle pedal. If it is too painful to complete a 360° cycle on the pedal then simply rock the pedal from side to side for a few days. There are many exercises that can be accomplished in a pool that again keeps the leg from bearing full weight. While gilding onto the side of the swimming pool, allow yourself to do gentle kicking but do this without letting your knee bend. This muscle contraction requires knee stability to increase the effectiveness of the water exercise. Others can include Aquatic Lateral Sweeping, as described on page 99, and Knee Lifts so that the water can give a small amount of friction resistance.

In the **Recovery phase,** include increasing the *FIT* of the Straight Leg raise by using ankle weights and doing more repetitions that are combined with maximum isometric contractions, when the knee is fully extended. Then starting the OSCP will preferentially activate and strengthen the VMO. In the latter part of the recovery phase you can also use a knee extension machine that has rollers to allow for free movement through the exercise, and do single repetitions when you are pain free in all movements and exercises. After all exercises can be done pain free, then use of the Smith Machine for free squats will be advantageous, and could be an exercise to use for continued knee health. The Smith Machine exercises were described in the previous section referring to *Patellofemoral pain syndrome*, and you may also use a leg extension sled as seen in picture 35.

<u>Knee Ligament Sprains & Tears Summary</u>
Acute Phase: FIRST 3 DAYS
  RICE
  Gentle Knee Flex/stretching
Rehab Phase: DAYS 4 TO 14
  Straight leg Raise
  Cycle for ROM, no resistance
  Water Exercise

Knee Ligament Sprains & Tears, Cont'd
Recovery: WEEKS 3 TO 6
Open Stance Cycling protocol
                Smith Machine squats
                Incline Leg extension sled

Meniscal Tears

Unfortunately, meniscal tears are injuries that are commonly not examined until they become a chronic source of pain and suffering. The symptoms of meniscal tears are similar to PFPS, and the symptoms include the following: pain from stairs, point-specific pain when exercising, "clicking" or *locking* of the joint in certain positions under weight, and meniscal tears also show excessive VMO atrophy.

The good news is that if an orthopedist diagnosed meniscal tears after using the McMurray movement test followed by MRI tests, then the arthroscopic trimming of the torn meniscal cartilage is a procedure with often the fastest recovery time of any orthopedic surgery. After Dr Spears accomplished the arthroscopic trimming of the author's torn meniscus, (not during the 16 post-crash operations), the author walked out of the surgical center after being discharged, and completed a full set of rehabilitation phases pain free. The design to follow could look like this, based on previously described exercises:

Meniscal Tear Post-operative Rehab Summary
Acute Phase: RICE
                (Expect excessive pain the first day)
                Cycle for ROM, no weight
Rehab Phase: Straight leg Raise
                Open Stance Cycling protocol
                Incline Leg extension sled
Recovery: OSCP
                Single Knee Extension mach
                Incline Leg Extension sled
                Smith Machine

93

Proactive Exercises for Knee Health

Unfortunately a population of people (particularly women) have a wide orthopedic alignment between their hip, knee, and tibia that predispose them for possible knee problems. This alignment is measured as the *Q-Angle,* and it is the angle between the line coming through the hip crest (Iliac crest) to the center of the knee cap (patella), and the second line of the angle is from the center of the patella to the ground. For all people who have suffered from knee injuries or chronic conditions, continual use of the exercises in the Recovery phases will benefit your overall knee health, and may be used proactively as well.

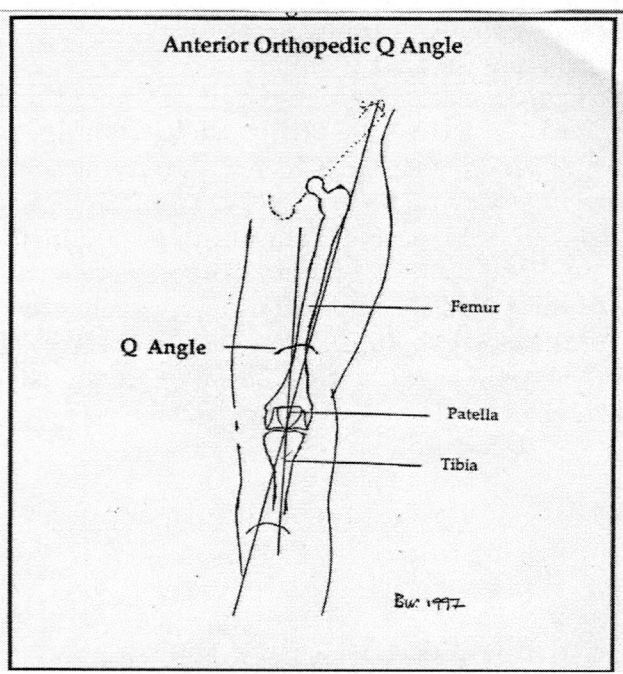

Figure #12 Anterior Q-Angle,

There have been many different exercise protocols described in these chapters and, one may question which is best to be a proactive exercise that helps reduce expected pain and/or symptoms. The answer to that question is based on a program's design for the same effective therapeutic steps, and those steps are: increased flexibility, increased blood flow, and muscular symmetry for increased strength.

Flexibility training exercises for the knee are utilized to stretch both the quadriceps, hamstring, and gracilius muscles. For the quadriceps stretching, one can accomplish this from a standing or supine position, (laying on a flat surface). Simply pull the heel towards the gluteus muscles for tension that achieves maximum knee flexion, which will flex Vastus Medialis Oblique, Vastus Lateralis, Sartorius, and Rectus Femoris. Variations may be accomplished by changing the position of the foot/ankle that is held in the stretch, and/or the exact direction that the ankle is pulled in adduction. Effective stretching techniques for the hamstrings and Gracilius have been described in earlier segments of this section.

For increased blood flow and activation/strengthening for muscular symmetry of VMO vs. VL, one should use the Open Stance Cycling Protocol (OCSP). This has been used effectively with symptomatic patients who have had many years of chronic knee pain and several different knee surgeries. There was a pilot study that examined the lasting effect of the OSCP for symptomatic patients, based on muscle activation while climbing and descending steps. A pilot study did show that training with the OSCP yielded continued, preferential VMO activation on the step tests. 3

Stretching and the OSCP could be an effective proactive exercise before situations that could be symptomatic, like extended seating, or in a situation where one may be standing still for long periods of time, or before climbing/descending many stairs. To test which protocol is the most effective and beneficial, one may use the same set of proactive protocols (i.e. four sets of stretches and 20 minutes on the OSCP at resistance level X on random resistance program). Then measure the pain/discomfort in these symptomatic settings on a scale of 1 to 11, and track the results. Then design the best combination for the best proactive exercise to avoid possible, expected pain or discomfort.

Other Exercises for the Knee include using elastic bands for resistance to knee extension and/or resistance for contracting or curling the knee. Accomplishing a hamstring curl on a prone machine slowly will also co-activate the knee stabilizer muscles. A more advanced exercise that is only appropriate for the recovery stage would be Plyometric jumps.

Plyometric exercises are ones that begin by lengthening of muscle, which is rapidly followed, by a shortening of the muscle (concentric contraction). Energy stored during the eccentric, lengthening phase is rapidly recovered by the subsequent concentric phase. When a high jumper runs towards the bar, the final action is to jump to a squat, which lengthens the quadriceps muscles, then the quadriceps concentric contraction is more powerful. This can be used as a final step after all pain has abated in all other exercise and the athlete wants to pursue further, more strenuous exercises.

LOWER LEG INJURIES

Shin Splint Syndromes

The term "Shin splints" is generally used to describe many pains of the lower leg, and many of these injuries are *overuse* injuries of the musculotendinous tissue covering the tibia. Upon feeling of acute pain in the back (posterior) of the leg bone, one must seek medical examination to insure that a stress fracture of the tibia has not occurred. This "shin splint" differs in the different region or compartment where pain is occurring, but the condition comes from three major sources:

  1) Unconditioned athlete attempting too vigorous training or sport, 2) Incorrect biomechanical positioning, such as improper position in the "runner starting blocks," and 3) Improper shoes which cause too large of a heel strike to be absorbed by the leg.

Symptoms then include pain, tenderness, occasional swelling of the inner part of the lower leg, tight calf muscles, and pain from toes radiated up the lower leg. In the *Acute phase* a unique treatment to follow the needed *RICE* is massage therapy. Since the dense musculotendinous tissue is hard to treat with increased blood flow and flexibility training, a deep tissue massage can be extremely helpful in the treatment of this condition.

The *Rehab phase* can begin with flexibility training for all of the major muscles in the lower extremities, i.e. quadriceps, hamstrings, gluteus, and gastrocnemius. The effective exercises will include non-impact cardiovascular training,(CV), such as on a stationary cycle or elliptical trainer, and this will yield increased blood flow to the musculotendinous tissue for repair. Stair climbing machines should be avoided because too often the biomechanical cause of this disorder has not been corrected yet, which means that the stair machines would yield painful symptoms, rather than rehabilitate this disorder. Also investigate and correct the various biomechanical components that could be contributing to and causing painful situations.

Recovery phase will have different durations than other injury therapies described, as the condition may take longer to heal. So interval time between training must be at least two complete days to ensure recovery of the musculotendinous tissue. Continue the flexibility and continue the non-impact cardiovascular training. Ice after the training activities will also help control the swelling and increase the recovery training benefits for the musculotendinous tissue. Light resistance training can be alternated with the cardiovascular training, but one must focus on slower concentric (muscle shortening) contractions rather than focusing on increasing the resistance used.

Shin Splint Syndromes, Rehab Summary

Acute Phase:	FIRST 3 DAYS
	RICE
	Massage Therapy
Rehab Phase:	DAY 3 to SECOND WEEK
	Flexibility Training
	Stationary Cycle
	Elliptical
	NO Stair Machines
Recovery:	WEEKS 3 to 6
	Training Intervals
	Bicycle Alternate Resistance

Calf Muscle Cramps

This condition has been associated with dehydration of athletes training in sports that require jumping and running. The old adage that an athlete should "eat salt" was used to prevent this disorder, since salt increases the fluid that the body is holding. We now know that increased salt invites prospective cardiovascular problems so ***athletes should never take salt tablets,*** but there are still three key steps that prevent cramps. The first is to drink water before, during, and after exercise or sport. Secondly a consistent, adequate warm up before exercise training prepares muscles for instant need for creatine in the fast twitch muscle activation, and cool down sessions will help reduce the "pooling" of lactic acid which contributes to cramps. [14,15,17] "Cool-down" is to reduce the intensity of the exercise but continue the motion or movement. For example, after performing many biceps exercise one should "cool-down" with

98

the curl action without weight, and a cool-down for knee training might be to ride the bicycle easily with no resistance inside.

The third component is to make sure that the athlete's diet is rich in mineral nutrients such as potassium and calcium.

Calf Muscle Cramps, Summary
Water before-during-after exercise
Warm up & Cool down stretching
Proper diet with RDA vitamins & minerals

Other strength training exercises for *Rehab* and *Recovery phases* of lower leg injuries would include: Aquatic Lateral Sweeping, Runner's Start training, Water Jumps, and Towel-Movement. The Aquatic Lateral Sweeping is done in a pool at chest depth water. Hold one hand on the side and sweep your outer leg away from your body as fast as you can, (Abduction). This can be done for 8 to 12 repetitions at the maximal power to be followed by 4-6 easy repetitions.

The runner's start exercise is simply to start from a sprint runner's position as if you were in the starting blocks and propel yourself out of the blocks as fast as possible. This should be a final exercise for the *Recovery phase*. The Water Jump exercise begins by standing chest deep in a swimming pool, and then one jumps up forcefully, but on the way down one will "curl up" to prevent any foot impact on the bottom of the pool.

The Towel-Movement exercise is to move or pull a towel by contracting your toes. Then manipulate the towel is different directions. Additional flexibility exercises for calf muscle cramps would include the Compass Direction movements of the foot/ankle, and Max squat stretches. To perform the compass direction training, start by moving your toes in the compass direction for increasing ROM. Start in a neutral position, then flex the foot up for north, and return to the neutral position. Then flex and rotate the foot to the right to mimic an easterly direction, followed by return to the neutral position, etc.

The max squat is simply to squat down as far as you can or until your buttocks reach your feet, while holding onto a

99

supportive structure. This should not be done with Achilles tendon injuries, but it does allow flexibility training for the foot and gluteus muscle and tendons.

FOOT-ANKLE INJURIES

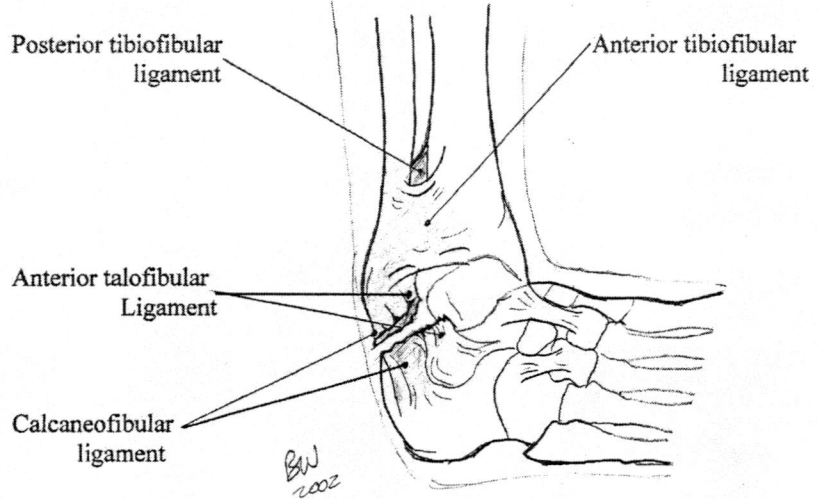

Posterior tibiofibular
ligament

Anterior tibiofibular
ligament

Anterior talofibular
Ligament

Calcaneofibular
ligament

Figure #13, Lateral Ankle Sprain

Lateral Ankle Sprain

A foot/ankle sprain is said to be the most common sports injury, and it is estimated that there is one ankle sprain per 10,000 Americans daily.[6,7,17] The lateral Ankle Sprain is actually a pull, stretch, or tear of the ligamentous connective tissue (Ligaments are the fibers that connect bone-to-bone.) Symptoms that often occur with ankle sprains can include any of the following: 1) A specific point that is tender or painful, 2) Ankle swelling, 3) Limping and pain when walking and/or standing, and 4) The inability to run or jump, 5) In severe sprains one would hear a "Pop" when the ankle injury occurred.

These symptoms make sense after one examines the ligaments that are damaged from a lateral hyperextension of the ankle, (or "rolling over" or "turning" your ankle), as seen in the illustration above. The treatment therefore should make sense in that you should immediately restrict movement and take action to reduce the swelling, inflammation, and pain

The *Acute Phase* of ankle injuries will begin with *RICE* (Rest, Ice, Compression, Elevation). An elastic bandage can be easily applied in a cross pattern. (Picture #43) Protection is imperative with a severe ankle injury and this may require immobilization with a cast or brace. If the sprain is not that severe, then one may only gently train your ROM. The Compression and Elevation are key for ankle rehab and recuperation after such an injury.

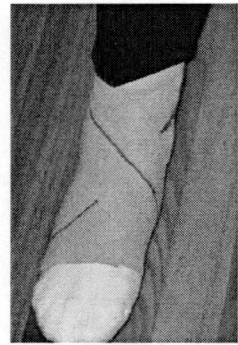

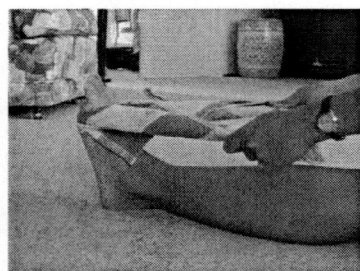

Pic #43 Elastic Bandage on Foot   **Pic #44** Ankle Flex-Stretch Towel

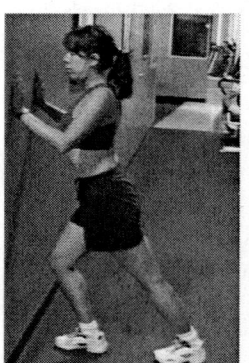

Pic #45 Runner's Stretch

Start the ***Rehab phase*** with further flexibility training and open-chained exercises. Since the foot has been injured, one should avoid closed-chained exercises (where one bears weight while the foot is in fixed contact with a surface). An elastic cable can be used effectively as light resistance in strengthening the muscles for plantar flexion and dorsi flexion. (Plantar flexion is pointing the ankle/toes down, and dorsi flexion is the opposite, upward movement). With a severe ankle injury, one should also work for free and complete movement of the toes. This is for rehabilitating the neuromotor control, as the nerve fibers may be injured with a major tear of the ankle ligament (calcaneofibular ligament).

Other open-chained exercises will include cycling when pain free and isometric contractions in association with the straight leg raise. Work in this phase to regain complete ROM. This is beneficial because in normal circumstances one uses all of these muscles in the coordination of walking and good flexibility with complete ROM may help prevent further ankle injuries. An exercise that is recommended for both strength training and neuromuscular control is the Foot Wobble Board. The wobble board can be purchased or made by anchoring a 2x2" board into the center of a piece of plywood that is 24" in diameter. (See picture #46)

Use this while seated and control the movement of the board with opposing muscle contraction. Rather than just pushing down your toes, which would make the wobble board tip to the floor, use a controlled movement of having it just rotate 15 degrees and return to a neutral position.

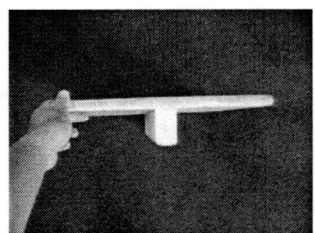

Pic #46, Wobble Board

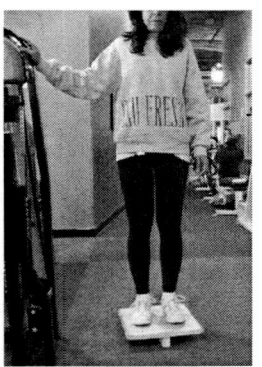

Pic #47, Standing on Wobble board

For *Recovery Training,* one may continue the coordinated muscular exercises with cycling, and an interesting additional exercise "Line Jumping," may be added only when the symptoms are no longer present and one is pain free, (Picture #48). Simply have both feet side-by-side and do the small but controlled jumps in a coordinated sequence. Strengthening of the calf muscles (Soleus and Gastrocnemius) can be accomplished by doing this. Calf muscle stretching (dorsi flexion) in a Runner's Stretch will be a tool you should perform before and after all activities from now on. (Picture #45) To stretch the main calf muscle (gastrocnemius), one should keep the knee fully extended, and to stretch the soleus, use the same position but keep the knee bent 10 - 15 degrees.

A Smith Squat machine will also help strengthen the unity muscular activation as needed in normal mobility. One should consider the frequency of the ankle sprains that occur because repeated problems could be an indication of a hyperelasticity disease.

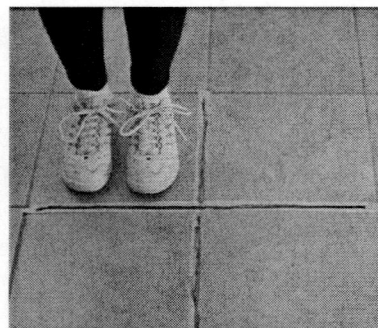

Pic #48 Line Jumping Start   →   Next Block

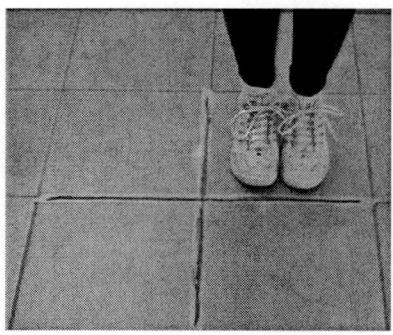

<u>Lateral Ankle Sprain, Rehab Summary</u>

Acute Phase: FIRST 3 DAYS
                 RICE + Crutches
                 ROM & Flexibility, **gently**

Rehab Phase: DAY 3 to SECOND WEEK
                 Flexibility training
                 Open-chained movement
                 Isometric contraction + SLR
                 Toe movement (neuromotor)
                 Seated Foot-Wobble-board
                 Cycle + calf muscle stretch

Recovery: WEEKS 3 to 6
                 Cycle + Flexibility training
                 Line jumping
                 Calf muscle strength training
                 Smith Squats

Heel/Sole Pain (Plantar Fasciitis)

Heel pain is common in many people, (particularly long distance runners), and the term "Plantar Fasciitis" is an umbrella term to describe chronic heel/foot pain. The Plantar Fascia is the connective tissue that links the muscular tissue to the heel on the sole of one's foot, and pain can be present in this area from many different causes. After pain is felt on the sole of one's foot, the injury's severity must be determined to ensure that it is not a calcaneal fracture or bone spur.

With this Plantar Fasciitis, the pain is often the worst when one gets out of bed in the morning, and diminishes after the foot/ankle has been *warmed up.* An acute, sharp pain can be present with increased weight bearing such as squatting heavy weights. People with this syndrome may be able to run and jump for short durations, but the condition will worsen if not treated.

The most effective treatments should include the insertion of a heel impact-absorbing, orthotic device. It has been found that a soft orthotic that can absorb the calcaneal impact force will help reduce the symptoms and reduce occurrence of plantar fasciitis. Using a small lift under the heel can reduce the stretching of the plantar fascia. [1,10] While this condition is most frequently chronic, it may have arisen from a repeated impact sport or activity, but it continues as an overload or repetitive stress injury.

The *Acute phase* treatment should include *RICE*, the use of crutches if needed or use of orthotic heel insert, and one should always avoid walking barefooted. While the duration of the treatment phases may differ greatly for each person, the order of protocols is still important. Soothing water therapy like soaking your foot in a tub of warm water can also be helpful in this phase because it will help increase the blood flow and relax the tissue.

The *Rehab phase* may begin effectively with flexibility training of the plantar fascicula, and this can be done by gently sliding the bottom of your foot over a rolling pin. This flexibility training should also be accompanied by strength training of the calf muscles (gastrocnemius and soleus), because inflexibility of those muscles may have played a significant role in the development of this disorder. The flexibility training in this stage might well be accomplished a towel or with elastic cords rather that standing against a wall as previously described.

As soon as the pain has abated, cardiovascular training is important because increased blood flow will help in the repair of the connective tissue. Isometric contractions of the calf muscles with plantar flexion and dorsi flexion positions will also be beneficial, in this phase as well.

A strength training exercise that can be made also into a cardiovascular exercise is Aquatic Lateral Sweeping, as described on page 99. This exercise is done with interval training (several repetitions at max effort followed by several easy repetitions. For this injury, continue doing this exercise of sweeping your leg away from you laterally while your other leg is beside the pool wall, for 20 straight minutes in chest-deep water. Alternate legs so that you are training your healthy leg as well to rest your fatigued injured leg, and to allow continuous, aerobic training at a slightly elevated heart rate. (For more information on techniques in aerobic, cardiovascular training see Chapter III.)

While performing exercises in the ***Recovery phase***, one needs to be conscious of benefit vs. risk, in continued actions that led to this condition in the first place. The orthotic should be worn every time one is walking after awaking each morning. Barefoot walking is a contributing factor to this disorder and Calcaneal bursitis. A unique strengthening exercise is Pool Jumping. Start in the swimming pool where the water is at chest depth, and bend the knees to prepare for a powerful jump upwards. Then jump as high out of the water as you can. The key ingredient though, is to land **without** touching the feet to the bottom of the pool. Extend your arms and curve your back after the jump so that the water absorbs all of the return impact force because landing on your feet will re-injure the plantar fascia. Cycling may also benefit this condition because there is no impact force and the seat of the bicycle bears your body weight rather than the foot. Isometric contractions may also benefit as a proactive exercise.

Plantar Fasciitis, Rehab Summary

Acute Phase: DAYS 1 TO 3

RICE

Orthotics

Aquatic Lateral Sweeping

Rehab Phase: DAYS 4 TO 14

Stretching (rolling pin)

Isometric contractions

Water Jumping

Recovery: WEEKS 3 TO 6

Pool Jumping,

(WITHOUT landing on your feet)

Stationary Cycling

Proactive Isometrics

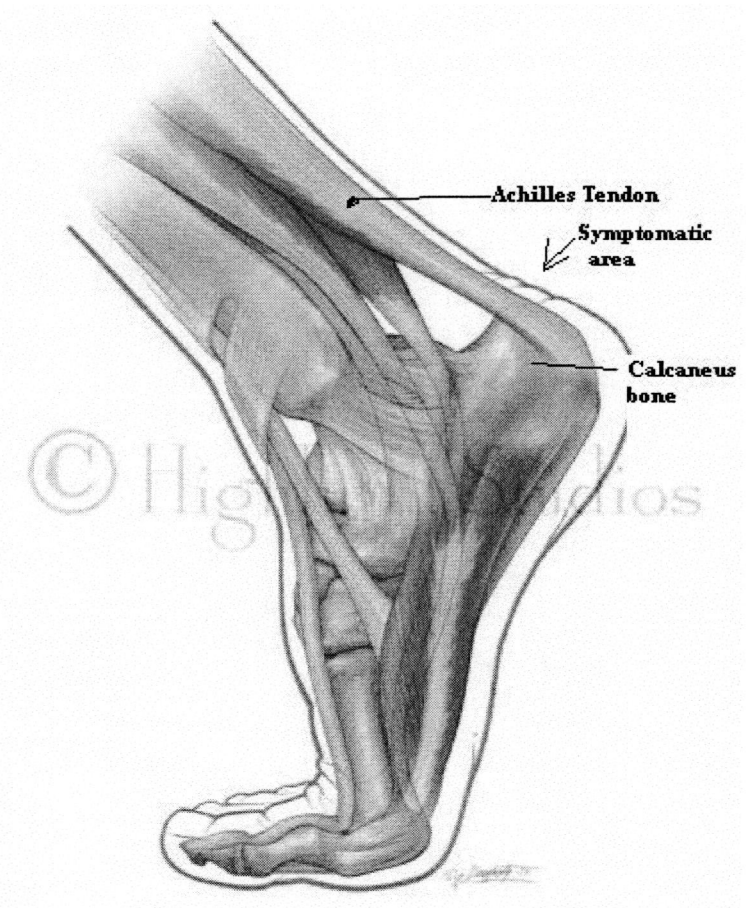

Figure #14, Foot/Ankle Musculature

Calcaneobursitis & Achilles Tendonitis

These are both common overuse injuries that have similar symptoms and require similar treatment. However, if one heard/felt a "Snap" or has acute pain in the area of the Achilles tendon it must be examined to ensure that a major tear or rupture has not occurred. A significant tear in the Achilles tendon will require surgical repair or it can lead to a lifelong disability.

Calcaneobursitis is inflammation of the bursa that surrounds the achilles tendon with insertion into the anklebone (calcaneus), and the arrow points to this area on figure #14.

Symptoms of calcaneobursitis include the following: Pain upon waking up in the morning, a quick, sharp pain when walking barefoot, and it has an identifiable "single-point" of pain. However, Achilles Tendonitis is a more gradual onset with increased pain coupled with decreased in ability to perform finely skilled foot movement (discrete motor functions such as moving the foot independent of leg movement). The Achilles tendon is the largest in the body, and treatment for both of these syndromes will be focused on flexibility training, reduction of impact force upon the heel, increased blood flow, and strengthening of the calf muscles, (gastrocnemius and soleus).

When the pain is acute, use the *Acute phase* protocol of *RICE* with an immobilization brace (having an elevated heel) to keep the Achilles tendon from being fully extended. Again, medical consultation is encouraged to identify the intensity of tendon damage and to prevent further rupture of the achilles tendon. An orthotic is effective for calcaneobursitis because the inflammation and pain begins at the tendon's insertion point.

The *Rehab phase* should be focused on flexibility training. There can be variation to the gastrocnemius and soleus stretching based on changes in foot position and knee flexion. A wobble board (Picture #46) is effective both for discreet motor training and neuromuscular coordination training, but one must start training with the wobble board while seated. Using flexibility training and the wobble board will help normalize the calf muscle activation (gastrocnemius), which is important for the health of the Achilles tendon. Begin the wobble board exercise while you are seated and when your pain has abated and you are stronger, then you may perform this exercise standing with a side support for safety (like doing this beside a pole or column that you can hold yourself steady on). Stationary cycling is effective without forcing the body to bear weight. It will increase the blood flow that is imperative for repair, and the increase in venous blood flow will reduce swelling. Indoor stationary cycling may even be accomplished while still wearing the immobilization brace to prevent excess lengthening of the achilles tendon. Again Aquatic Lateral Sweep training would be beneficial

Recovery phase requires further flexibility training, which should be done as a daily, proactive treatment. A unique strengthening exercise is to accomplish single leg standing that can also be beneficial for optimizing neuromuscular control of the entire single leg. The "Heel lift" exercises for the calf muscle (gastrocnemius) training may be varied for focus on concentric contraction. To accomplish this, focus on lifting the heel while isometrically contracting the other leg muscles. Then relax all muscles as the heel comes down.

On other days, one may alternate by focusing on the eccentric contractions (muscle lengthening), and letting the heel drop more slowly, under conscious muscular control. Stationary cycling should also be continued during this phase and as proactive exercises in the future.

<u>Calcaneobursitis & Achilles Tendonitis</u>
<u>Rehab Summary</u>
Acute Phase: RICE
      (Orthotics for Calcaneobursitis)
      (Immobilization with elevated heel
      for Achilles tendonitis)
Rehab Phase: Flexibility training
      seated Wobble Board
      Cycle training
      Aquatic Lateral Sweep
Recovery: Single Leg stance
      Alternating heel raise
      Cycle + Flexibility training

Chapter V
Design and Follow the Rehabilitation Program

Designing your Rehab Program

Now that you have seen all of the components that are frequently used in rehabilitation programs, and you have seen clinical examples for common orthopedic injuries, it is time to design your own program. Beginning your exercise therapy without a specific design may leave you with too many plateaus or if you're over eager, your efforts may be too aggressive or too fast, causing further injury. Remember that once your pain, inflammation, and swelling have been reduced, you want to focus your plan conservatively enough so that these symptoms do not reoccur. The primary objectives of your program should include:

1. Safety
2. Increased blood flow
3. Regain Range of motion (ROM)
4. Restore complete neuromuscular control
5. Counteract muscle atrophy
6. Regain and increase strength and power
7. Regain and increase endurance for sport and normal activities
8. Safety

The injury analysis and the rehab *Phases* are integral components that must be interwoven for a successful program design. As you read the clinical components and examples in Step IV, you may have seen the outline of your program, but each person has a different speed and different goals. One must immediately treat the injury's pain, inflammation, and swelling before anything else, and this is accomplished in the *Acute phase* of rehab. Once that has been accomplished and the pain is under control, then you can design your program for your short-term and long-range goals. Plan your program and follow the plan!

Allow yourself extra time or be prepared for extra challenges because your body may respond differently to the rehab therapies discussed in chapter IV. The *Acute phase* is beneficial to follow because those phases are safe, conservative, but they are challenging enough to decrease muscle atrophy. The old phrase "No pain no gain" is wrong! Your body sends you pain messages about damage or potential damage. So pushing yourself harder each week **before** you feel pain is good but pushing beyond pain can cause serious, secondary injuries when you are in rehabilitation.

If the injury was acute enough to require medical care then the professionals should be happy to discuss your rehabilitation with you, and let your healthcare professional know that you are using this book. The more involved you are in active pursuit of your rehab goals, the more likely you are to obtain those goals at the fastest pace possible. Set goals for all of the small steps and remember that many small steps can climb the mountainous challenge of orthopedic rehabilitation. I hope you find each step more exciting and that each step makes you more eager for further success.

If you follow one of the exercise therapies, you should still begin with the initial testing and track all of your progress. As you come to the *Rehab phase*, you may need to add different exercise or stretches. You can choose additional exercises from the lists at the end of Step III, and each stretch or strength training exercise is explained in the close of each section of exercise therapy. (For example the stretching protocol "Knee tuck" is described in the closing section of *Hip, thigh injuries.*)

F.I.T.

We have described the use of Frequency, Intensity, and Time (or duration) of exercise previously, but *F.I.T.* must be used and included for planning your exercise therapy. While it is inappropriate to say before beginning that on "Day *X*, I will increase the intensity," it is also important that you allow for variation in your rehab schedule.

Changes in *F.I.T.* allow one to gradually increase the difficulty level of the exercise or training whether that is strength training, flexibility training, plyometric training, or aerobic, cardiovascular training. For example when using an exercise therapy for a knee disorder, there will become times that you need to make each exercise more difficult, so that you continue increasing in strength. So rather than going immediately from squatting zero weight on the Smith Machine® to squatting 200 lbs, one will need many subtle, slight increases or changes (in more than just changing the weight)

So plan, and literally write into your program that at your next progression to be increased Frequency (more repetitions) or Intensity (a little more weight OR a lower squat). Plan ahead that your third progression would be to increase the total Time with squatting on the Smith Machine® by adding another set. Plan the subtle progression, and make that progression gradually with *FIT* to help you benefit more completely from using a designed program. That complete benefit will be a stronger joint that is less likely to be injured in the future, (or it won't be easily injured).

Modifying existing programs

If your injury is not listed in the exercise therapies of common injuries, then find the example that is closest to your injury. Next, follow the *Acute phase* as close as possible with safety first. You may alter the rehab design if exercises in the *Rehab phase* are too demanding or if you need more challenging exercises. As I advised that safety should be your first concern, it is often advisable to add extra stretching protocols before adding additional strength training exercises.

Design your rehab plan and plan to follow your design.

Self Medicating with Activity of Enjoyment

A unique concept that many healthcare providers miss, is helping you find out what activities can bring you the emotional and athletic joy while you are in rehab. I learned of this from a friend, Patch Adams MD, and he has been one of my mentors who has helped me focus my efforts towards medical *Service.* As a competitive athlete in bodybuilding and power lifting, my greatest emotional challenge from the traumatic plane crash was the forced immobilization of my legs. Inactivity for me was the toughest obstacle, and getting the chance to train again was fun. My many surgeons, particularly Ted Spears MD, understood and empathized with my need to "move freely," and because he understood, he gave me the tools, advice, and ideas that would help me enjoy my rehab.

It was a very exciting day when I was first able to stand upright again (even though I was still wearing casts on both legs from toe to hip). I had tremendous difficulty even standing after 6 months of being restricted to a wheelchair and the resulting muscle atrophy (decrease in muscle mass, that had resulted in my losing over 50 lbs of muscle weight). So just being upright was my first *Activity of Enjoyment!*

As my rehabilitation from wheelchair movement to using a walker progressed, I relished the Physical Therapy rehab because it felt like another fun athletic challenge for me. Each rehab session, my PT would ask me what I wanted to achieve for the day, and I would work to do just a little more than I had previously accomplished. My answer would be like "Ok I'll do 5 laps around the hospital today!" That was a long way from the 485lbs that I had squatted the month before my plane crash, but I truly felt blessed that God had given me another chance to start afresh and work for better results each day!

Activities that help with pain

What activities help you feel better, happy, and recharge your emotional batteries? You must find the activities that help you turn your mind away from pain, even for just a short time, and this will be an effective respite from your pain that will help excel your recovery.

Bicycling was the favorite activity that helped me through the 3 years of: Operations - followed by rehab - to be followed again by the next operation (this was the sequence for many of the 16 operations). I was doing my own rehab work at that time for two reasons. First, I knew my body and I knew the rehab protocols to follow under the guidance of my surgeon, physician, and friend, Ted Spears MD. A complete team effort requires the participation of the patient too. Second, my major medical insurance had expired after the first 30 days in neural ICU after the plane crash, so all of the later operations, hospitalization, and rehab were true gifts from my caring providers. TYG!

I felt stronger and more active when I was on the bicycle, and with Dr. Spears permission, I was regularly on the bicycle the day after most operations for a low intensity, morning ride. This activity was beneficial for me physically (because of the increased blood flow, neuromuscular control, and strengthening), but bicycling was tremendously powerful for me emotionally. It was a true joy to have the speed of movement again, and to be working on my rehab progression! I have to admit that I loved seeing the amazed look on people's faces in San Marcos, Tx when they saw me bicycling past them – wearing a cast! One time when I was cycling in a blue foot/ankle brace, I heard a little boy tell his Mother, "Mom I want a fast boot like that!" This feeling of excitement and joy helped block out the pain, while I was bicycling, and it was enough of a respite from the constant pain that it helped me go throughout the rest of my day.

Other activities that have been reported to help people in similar ways are as follows: [17]
- Horseback Riding
- Activity with children
- Watching movies
- Dancing
- Swimming
- Sitting by the ocean side
- Reading to Children
- Humor
- Water Aerobics
- Painting
- Sculpting

Most any activity that does not injure you can be effective to give you a respite from your pain, and in my experience with bicycling, that activity yielded increased secretion of endorphins and catecholamines, which block or subdue the pain signals.

Cardiovascular training and endorphin secretion

Endorphins are secreted by the Anterior Pituitary gland in response to stress of different levels. [1,2,16,22] The secretion is increased with longer duration(s) of exercise like aerobic, cardiovascular exercises that last over 20 minutes. This could have been an effective tool for humans several hundred years ago, because if one needed to flee a threat and run for 30 minutes the endorphins would help keep the pain subdued so that the person could get away. One might be able to use such an activity like cardiovascular exercise training to get away from the pain.

The catecholamines (epinephrine and norepinephrine) are hormones secreted by the adrenal glands and are considered "fight or flight" hormones because they assist the body's functioning during exercise. The catecholamines cause increased heart rates, increased heart stroke volumes (the amount of blood pumped out in each beat), increased blood vessel constriction, decreased gastral motility, and thereby increases the body's ability to fight or flee. [23,24] The catecholamines help the body's ability to use all energy for exercise and to diminish most extraneous functions that would deter exercise such as bowel movements, joint restriction, and/or pain.

True cardiovascular training is endurance training (over 20 minutes) where one has a stable, elevated heart rate of 70 – 75% of one's maximal heart rate. To calculate your "target heart rate" you subtract your age from 220, (This is the estimated maximum heart rate that your body could obtain at your age). Multiply that number by .70 or 70% to get your "target heart rate" for aerobic cardiovascular exercise. Cardiovascular exercise needs to be 20 minutes or more for lipid consumption, but the same exercise that last over 12 minutes will have the effect of endorphin and catecholamine secretions. [22,24] Any exercise that yields a consistently elevated heart rate will be an effective exercise to help you have a respite from pain, as long as it does not complicate your injury or worsen it. The following are popular modes of CV training:
- Bicycling
- Swimming
- Water Aerobics

- Circuit training
- Speed Walking
- Running
- Arm cycling
- Aerobic dancing
- Cross Robics
- Stair climbing (Stair Master machines)
- Elliptical training (equipment similar to cross country skiing)

Once again your rehabilitation should be a team effort. If you are under the care of a healthcare provider, consult with your team as to which exercise mode might benefit you the most in this area.

Chapter VI
Goal Analysis & Completion

You began the *Second Step* in your rehabilitation by testing your Range of Motion, Flexibility, Strength, and Endurance. So check your progression by repeating those same tests every few weeks. Measure the degree of flexibility and extension, and measure your range of motion. Then for *strength testing*, you should measure this in a repeatable way that measures exactly your maximum strength *before* pain erupts.

Testing

If you do not have pain when you are exercising, then you may measure your One Repetition Maximum, (1RM). This is the largest amount of weight or tension that you can lift in the exercise to be tested. Before testing your 1RM, start with stretching to be followed by movement with only a very light weight to gain increased blood flow to the area of exercise. For instance, before I squat my 1RM, I stretch and then begin with a few repetitions without weight, only the bar. That helps me *warm up* my motion for the squat, and then I may just use a little weight to prepare my muscles for their maximum effort. After that preparation, I attempt my previous 1RM, or in most cases I attempt a slightly higher weight than I have been able to lift previously. If I have success at this weight, then after resting a minute or two, I will attempt a higher weight for my new 1RM.

If you were not able to reach your desired 1RM, then rest and settle for attempting a lower weight to be your max on this day. The more your attempt your 1RM, the more fatigued you will be and, there are many independent variables that can effect the performance of your maximal effort, such as diet, sleep, pre-exercise activity, etc. Don't think badly of yourself if your performance was not on the level that you desired. As in power-lifting, before you test the next time, accomplish several weeks of regular exercise, and terminate all training two days before your next 1RM test. Make sure that you sleep for 10 hours, on each of the two nights before your lift. Then shoot for the best, but be happy hat you have come this far!

For endurance tests, use the same protocol and technique(s) that you used initially. For example if you are testing your endurance on a Lifecycle® you must make sure that you have the same seat height, the same program selected, and the same resistance, so that it can be an effective test of measuring *apples vs. apples.*

Progression

This might be an appropriate time to examine how close you are to reaching your goals. Compare your status to the tasks that you performed when you originally set your goals. There were five primary tasks you were to complete in setting your goals for rehabilitation, and those tasks included:
- Writing down your ultimate goal
- Noting performance goals
- Have others noticed you reaching or progressing towards your goal
- Progress charting
- Short term goal completion(s)

Alterations

Where are you in progress to completing your ultimate goals? Have you set new short-term goals, and how is your progress advancing? These are questions that you should ask yourself twice a month so that you are recalling the condition of your injury when you began your rehabilitation and the condition that you are in now along this pathway.

Now might be a good time to examine the program that you have designed or have followed in this book. If you have reached a certain level of performance but are no longer progressing, then it may be time to start new or additional exercises in your *Recovery phase* exercises. For this note the additional exercises listed in the closure of each common orthopedic injury in Chapter IV, and the complete list of strength training and flexibility exercises are in Chapter III. Challenge yourself and experiment with changes in your *Recovery* phase training so that you can reach your goal or get to an even higher performance.

Completion

When will your rehab training be complete? You set your goals in the second *Step,* and once you have met your goal, you can focus on higher goals. Using *Steps* in working towards other physical goals should help you as it has helped other people like the nurse who went from a traumatic head injury to completing in triathlons. Just make sure that you don't limit yourself to the exercises and protocols listed in this book. There are many different exercises, techniques, and training protocols for the different sporting or recreational events that exceed the rehab protocols in this book.

As you pursue goals beyond the specific goals that you set after your injury, make sure to include gradual progression with *F.I.T.* so that your efforts will pay off. If you have another injury remember *R.I.C.E.* and that will be an effective initial treatment for most non-traumatic injuries.

"Proactive" can be defined as performing action(s) that can help prevent or diminish an unpleasant, expected pain, which occurs due to a physical ailment. For example, a person with a knee injury or disorder, frequently has pain from long durations being seated in one place (frequently called "Stadium seating syndrome"). So a proactive exercise would be the exercise(s) done before being seated for a long time that would diminish or alleviate the expected knee pain.

Proactive exercises for arthritic and sports injury conditions are exercises that have continual movement but include varied or random resistance for the maximal blood flow to the muscle and fatigue of both the slow twitch and fast twitch muscle fibers of the symptomatic joint(s). For the greatest effect one should start with stretching, use an effective proactive exercise for muscle fatigue and blood flow (for 20 minutes or more), and complete your proactive session with cool down stretching. The next section offers proactive protocols designed for the areas of injuries addressed in Chapter IV.

Proactive Exercises

Proactive protocols will be described following the *region's name*. An effective proactive protocol for *foot/ankle* disorders (after stretching) would include riding an indoor bicycle with a random or interval resistance program. Then one should alternate stretching and maximal isometric contractions as the injury allows, for as long as feasible. An optimal proactive sequence would begin with pre exercise stretching, then 30 minutes of riding, followed by 15 minutes of isometric contractions (muscle contractions without moving the limb) and post exercise stretching.

Riding an indoor, computerized bicycle (such as the Lifecycle®), or using an elliptical trainer with interval programming would be helpful proactive exercises for _knee disorders._ One should avoid a stair machine for proactive treatment because the shear force of stepping can aggravate many knee disorders, and pain from stair climbing is also a common symptom of many knee disorders. [1,2,6,10,12]

Proactive exercises for _Hip/Thigh_ injuries will vary because of the very different injuries that range from sartorius sprain (deep quadriceps muscle) to hamstring tears (biceps femoris). The symptoms are very different but the proactive premise is the same. If you can find an exercise(s) that is continual, and also works your primary muscles to fatigue, then that exercise should be proactively effective for you. For example, people with hip injuries following "hip fractures" of the greater trochanter bone (which extends from the top of the femur), often have atrophy of the pelvic muscles. This causes pain and problems from long durations standing or long durations seated. An effective proactive protocol for this specific disorder is to use an elliptical machine with random resistance program, and you should attempt full range of leg motions, (based on your leg length).

Two exercises that are commonly used proactively for _Lower Back Pain_ (LBP) are the rowing machine, the elliptical machine with arm attachments, and abdominal crunches. This requires the same components of muscle fatigue and blood flow, and blood flow is even more important for this area because the lumbar disk degeneration is a symptom of LBP syndrome. [14,15,24] Start with flexibility training (described on page 23), and one of the proactive exercises described. Then perform as many abdominal crunches as you can, to be followed by cool-down with post-training stretching.

The _shoulder and thoracic back_ have a large number of exercises to choose from, but the best proactive option would be to combine 4 to 6 exercises in a circuit, to fatigue the muscle while keeping an elevated heart rate for increased blood flow. Obviously this takes a lot of equipment and planning so a training facility would be the best location for this, but imagination can make this accessible at home too. A true "Circuit Set" of training is a series of exercises, followed one right after another, without stopping which yields an elevated heart rate for aerobic training plus strength training resulting in muscular fatigue. To do this you have to set up each station in advance so that you can move fluidly through all of the exercises without stopping. If you are at a training facility, then simply plan the equipment to be used and walk quickly when changing machines. An example of this as a proactive "Circuit Set" for shoulder and upper back would be the 3 continuous sets, as follows:

- Butterfly DB, Elbow Abduction: 14 – 15 reps (pg. 56)
- Dumbbell Pectoral Fly exercise: 14 – 15 reps (pg. 61)
- Latissimus Dorsi Pull down: 14 – 15 reps (pg. 61)
- Military Press: 14 – 15 reps (described on pg. 60)

- Butterfly DB, Elbow Abduction: 14 – 15 reps
- Dumbbell Pectoral Fly exercise: 14 – 15 reps
- Latissimus Dorsi Pull down: 14 – 15 reps
- Military Press: 14 – 15 reps

- Butterfly DB, Elbow Abduction: 14 – 15 reps
- Dumbbell Pectoral Fly exercise: 14 – 15 reps
- Latissimus Dorsi Pull down: 14 – 15 reps
- Military Press: 14 – 15 reps

To complete this proactive routine, one would continuously proceed through all of the exercise sets without rest or with only very little rest between sets (no more than 120 seconds rest between sets). In a circuit, each "Set" is each group of four exercises. The cadence for completing each exercise would be a smooth, non-rushed repetition of one rep for every two seconds. For example starting with the Butterfly DB, Elbow Abduction, you would begin slightly bent over with the dumbbells held together in front of you. (See Picture #17, page 57.) The beginning movement where you separate the dumbbells and extend your elbows out (abduction) should take a full second (count "one thousand and one"), and then returning your elbows to the starting position (ergonomic movement of muscle lengthening) should also take one full second.

Proactive training for the _elbow_ may require a different approach because elbow pain is most frequently felt in sporting activities such as golf, tennis, and bowling. For these activities

123

the proactive steps would be to accomplish three sets of three different elbow stretch exercises before and after the athletic event (See page 64-65). If one has much elbow movement in another past time such as flying or directing an orchestra, then effective, proactive exercises would be to stretch, and then do the Winding/Unwinding exercise for 10 minutes straight, to be followed by another three sets of three different stretching protocols. An alternative to the winding exercise could be bar curls and reverse curls or the arm ergonometric exercise that were described on page 68.

Proactive exercise and needs for _wrist_ pain is very similar to elbow. Use the same techniques of stretching with muscle fatigue and increased blood flow. Exercises that can be done continuously for 10 – 12 minutes for this would be the wrist curl and reverse wrist curl that would be used with pre and post stretching.

Alternative, effective therapies/techniques/equipment

The alternative therapeutic techniques and modalities described below can be effective but must only be performed by educated, licensed professionals. This list of protocols are listed to inform you of the risks, benefits, and precautions that should be associated with each alternative therapy.

Ultrasound therapy involves a machine that generates sound waves of high speed (over 20,000 cycles per second), and this yields a vibration that is transferred through your muscle and or connective tissue. Heat therapy is often used to precede the ultrasound, and this makes sense because one should avoid vigorously activating muscles and connective tissue until the tissue is "warmed up." The benefit of ultrasound is increased blood flow to an injured area that may not be suitable for exercise therapy yet, and it yields decreased pain and muscular relaxation in areas treated. This may seem similar to the result of having a good, relaxing massage.

One should not use the instrument around areas that could be easily damaged by such high frequency action, such as the head, eye, spine, uterus (when pregnant or trying to become pregnant), all other reproductive organs, and open wounds. The intensity of the signal should not be too high.

Massage Therapy should only be performed by a Registered, Licensed Massage Therapist who has specialized training in sports medicine. You should investigate the background of your massage therapist to ensure that their assistance will benefit you as much as possible. The benefits of massage therapy are increased blood flow, relaxed muscles, and reduction of muscle tetany (which is constant, repeated muscle activation on a lower scale than a muscle spasm), and massage therapy also helps the body work to reabsorb excess lactic acid that is secreted in response to intense anaerobic exercise. Massage therapy can be beneficial, but you must communicate to the massage therapist about your injury, about any areas that you wish to be avoided, and tell your massage therapist when anything hurts.

Caution should be taken with inflamed areas that should benefit more from ice than the increased blood flow of massage. Massage therapy should be avoided over any open wounds, so that the structural repair that your body is doing does not become destroyed and because the lotion or cream that is used could potentially infect your wound.

Electrotherapy is often used as an initial post operative treatment because the alternating current of electricity that is transmitted through the electrodes to your muscles cause contractions in varying degrees where exercise would be detrimental or impossible at this time. Electrotherapy keeps the muscles active to decrease muscle atrophy (decrease in muscle size), it works to deter muscle spasms, and electrotherapy effectively increases blood flow, thereby increasing tissue healing. A Physical Therapist who has had extensive training with this equipment (such as a *TENS,* muscular stimulation unit), will greatly help your recovery by using this equipment.

However, one should always be cautious and question each person's training with this equipment, otherwise it can be very damaging. Too often unlicensed, untrained undergraduate college students who work in physical therapy clinics may be administering this treatment, and you should not allow this to happen to you. The danger of electrotherapy is that is can cause severe neural muscular signal transduction if applied in the wrong area at too high a voltage intensity. It should never be used around open wounds or healing fractures. It should never be used around sensitive areas to include the eyes, head, heart, reproductive organ areas, herniated disks, and it should never be used around the orthopedic growth plates of children or adults.

Heat modalities are effectively used, and this is a treatment that you can use at home with a heating pad if your health professional advises you. The superficial heating is done in clinics with water packs, and one should use caution when using an electrical "heating pad" at home. Most home devices (heating pads and hot water bottles) do not have a constant temperature or one that can be specifically altered to fit your needs as can be done with clinical equipment. The benefits of heat modalities are increased blood flow and preparation for exercise therapy or further treatment, and the effect is a more relaxed muscular tissue.

The temperature that is right for your needs is more complex and more dangerous than one might guess. For instance people who have circulatory problems have a higher risk for burns with this treatment. This therapy should also not be used in areas of decreased neural sensation for the same reason in avoiding burns. It should not be used over areas that have been treated for reduced pain, so avoid heat therapy over localized anesthetics for at least 48 hours after treated. People who have hemophilia, diabetes, or any similar conditions should avoid this treatment all together, and heat should never be used over areas of inflammation.

Hydrotherapy can ,mean Aquatic, kinetic (movement) therapy that can be done in swimming pools and it is also a term for specialized medical treatment to cleanse open wounds. The latter is designed for a more acute, severe injuries. Aquatic, kinetic therapy is very beneficial as an initial, conservative treatment because it can yield increased blood flow, it allows treatment of areas with reduced weight-bearing, and it allows effective resistance therapy that respects each person's different limits, more than a simple "chosen weight" on a machine would do. (Kinetic means "movement"). This is also an effective, continued *Recovery phase* treatment for many different injuries. The safety of this modality is so beneficial in a pool that is waist or chest deep, and it has few disadvantages.

There should always be another person present while you are training in the water (such as a lifeguard or physical

126

therapist), because muscle cramps or unexpected, acute pain can make a person drown in shallow water.

Benefits of Regular Exercise

Since you are reading this book, you probably have a regular pattern of exercise or a sport that you participate in. However, if you are not regularly exercising, then this section may help you or may help you advise someone else. "Regular exercise" is defined as exercise that substantially increases one's heart rate, continuously for over 20 minutes, three times a week, or participating in strength training exercise (resulting in muscular fatigue), lasting over 30 minutes. [22,32,34] So golf, bowling, and fishing are great sports and activities, but they are not in the category of "beneficial, therapeutic exercise."

In 1996 the US Surgeon General made the public proclamation that "Lack of Exercise is bad for one's health,." This was based on a large-scale, longitudinal study that showed such substantial findings that the Surgeon General reported the following:

"Regular physical activity that is performed on most days of the week reduces the risk of developing or dying from some of the leading causes of illness and death in the United States. Regular physical activity improves health in the following ways:
- Reduces risk of dying prematurely
- Reduces the risk of dying from heart disease
- Reduces the risk of developing diabetes
- Reduces the risk of developing high blood pressure
- Helps reduce blood pressure in people who already have high blood pressure
- Reduces the risk of developing colon cancer
- Reduces depression and anxiety
- Helps control weight
- Helps to build and maintain healthy bones, muscles, and joints
- Helps older adults become stronger and better able to move about without falling
- Promotes psychological well-being" [31]

Illnesses prevented or benefited by regular exercise

Osteoporosis is the bone disease where the bone tissue density is decreased by decreased bone deposition, and this is combined with increased bone breakdown to free Calcium (osteoclastic activity). [24,25,26] ("Freeing calcium" is the cellular breakdown of bone tissue which increased the Calcium in the blood.) This disease is more prominent in postmenopausal women, but it does occur in a significant number of men. The causes for osteoporosis include the following:

1. Lack of stress or muscle tension upon the bones
2. Malnutrition in decreased Calcium and decreased vitamin D intake or absorption
3. Lack of vitamin C (needed for bone deposition)
4. Postmenopausal decreased Estrogen, (needed for stimulating bone deposition)
5. Old age
6. Cushing's syndrome (substantial decrease in protein deposition)

Osteoporosis, understandably is a condition that frequently includes skeletal rigidity with frequent falls and fractures. [24,25] Weight bearing exercises are needed to reduce the losses in bone mass density (BMD) for many post menopausal women. While exercise is not the only treatment for this disease it is the primary, preventative exercise that can help prevent the disease from erupting. This is because the muscle's and/or tendon's pull on the bones causes a following reaction of modifying the bone to better handle that load when it is repeated. This is osteoblastic "Building" and deposition of bone tissue.

Conditions with decreased Bone Mass Density (BMD) can be treated by the following: Weight bearing exercise routines, Calcium and vitamin D supplements, Hormone replacement therapy (when test results show deficiencies), Flexibility training, Cardiovascular Exercise, Coordination exercises (also reduces the risk of falls and fractures), and by stopping smoking. Following these prescribed treatments should allow one to

128

regain a healthy skeleton, and terminate the bone tissue losses. [24,25,26,27]

High Blood pressure or Hypertension is defined as blood pressure that is higher than 140/90. It has been estimated that as many as 17% of the American population may be afflicted with hypertension, and it has also been shown that hypertension increases a person's risk of death by cardiovascular heart disease (CVHD) by up to 300%. [22,24,27, 28] This difficult problem can be prevented with aerobic, cardiovascular training because cardiovascular training works to increase the elasticity in the blood vessels and to deter the onset of this disease, and/or effectively treat the disease. This has been shown conclusively in many recent studies, and the blood has been significantly decreased in as little as three weeks. Unfortunately when the subjects in the tests discontinued their aerobic training, their blood pressure went back up. [22,24,27, 28]

There are many different independent variables that contribute to this disease, such as excess body weight (more than 20% over your ideal body weight), inactivity, and genetic predisposition. These variables are also helped with aerobic, cardiovascular training, and this can effectively decrease the mortality expected with this disease.

Type II Diabetes Mellitus, or *Non-insulin dependant diabetes* is a condition where the receptors of insulin are not effectively sensitive to the adequate supply of insulin in the body (frequently called "Insulin resistance.") This deters the breakdown of glucose (molecular sugars), resulting in blood glucose levels to be over 140mg/dl. People with this disease though, can also benefit greatly from aerobic, cardiovascular exercise. [24] Aerobic, cardiovascular exercise benefits people with Type II Diabetes by reducing their weight and body fat, and also by increasing their activity level. It has also been suggested that the increased fat utilization seen in diabetes can be beneficially changed with cardiovascular training for a decrease in one's blood/glucose levels.

Cancer is a general term for uncontrolled, excessive cell growth in the body. There are over 120 different types of cancer, and in the year 2000, the NIH National Cancer Institute study revealed that over 60,000 deaths that year were attributed to cancer. [35] Several epidemiological studies and exercise physiology studies have shown that exercise yields a significant

129

reduction in the risk of cancer. [22,29,30] The effects of regular exercise include increased levels of lymphokines (cells that are integral in production of antibodies) and other mechanisms that also help decease cancer occurrence in the human body. Regular aerobic, cardiovascular exercise has even been shown to be beneficial in treating breast cancer. There have even been powerful studies, such as one with over 30,000 subjects that have shown regular exercise to "Prevent breast cancer." This study went even further showing that daily exercising was better than exercising just 2-3 times per week. Increased exercise frequency substantially decreased the "Occurrence rate" of breast cancer for women in this study. [30]

Cardiovascular Heart Disease (CVHD) patients benefit significantly from exercise therapy, and it has been shown that exercise helps prevent onset of these diseases. [22,24] CVHD includes many different disorders that include the following:

1) Diseases of the heart muscle (Myocardial infarction, Angina, and Pericarditis)
2) Diseases of the valves (Mitral valve prolapse, endocarditis, and stenosis)
3) Diseases of the cardiac, neural conduction (Arrhythmias, Tachycardia, and Bradycardia)
4) Vascular artery and vein disease (Arthrosclerosis).

Because of the wide variety of problems in CVHD, the exercise therapy cannot have one benefit that affects all of these anomalies. Exercise though does prevent CVHD, and it effectively helps in the recovery of CVHD onset, through professional cardiac rehabilitation. One needs a full examination for the appropriate exercise prescription for each type of cardiovascular heart diseases, but the appropriate exercise prescription can halt the progress, onset, and eventual death from CVHD.

Even people who have pulmonary disorders such as emphysema, cystic fibrosis, and asthma can also benefit from cardiovascular exercise training. However, this training must be carefully prescribed and monitored so that constant attention is given to the patient and attention to the intensity of the training. The goal for training people with pulmonary disorders is to increase the efficiency of the gas exchange in breathing for a greater oxygen saturation of arterial blood. As a side effect, this training also improves patients' functional abilities and decreases shortness of breath.

Regular exercise is beneficial in many different realms that include: Proactively decreasing arthritic pain, Helping avoid life-threatening illness, and rehabilitation from orthopedic injuries or disease. The seven steps that were used in designing effective orthopedic rehabilitation will work well for many different physical challenges that benefit from exercise. The *Seven Steps* are:

I Injury Analysis
II Setting Rehab Goals
III Determine the Components for Rehab Success
IV Examine the Current Exercise Therapies
V Design and Follow your own Rehabilitation Program
VI Measure Progress and Determine Completion of Goals & Rehab
VII Proactive Exercises and Lifestyle Fitness

The last bit of advice that I want to share is to encourage you to enjoy the challenge of your rehabilitation. It might be easy for lots of people to be sad and depressed by their injuries (whether it be a sprained ankle of traumatic injury), but optimism and always looking ahead rather than behind, really works! Take the time to investigate the options for your rehabilitation, and then . . . Design your rehab plan and plan to follow your design!

So have fun in your rehab, and as the Pilot in me says,
"Kick the Tires, Light the Fires, and
I'll see you on the horizon!"

References, suggested readings

1. Kibbler WB, Herring SA, Press JM. *Functional Rehabilitation of Sports and Musculoskeletal Injuries*, Bolinas California, Aspen Publications, 1998
2. Canavan. *Rehabilitation in Sports Medicine*
3. Willis B, Burkhardt E, Walker J, Johnson M, and Spears T. "Patellofemoral Strength Training," Chapter 8, Knee Disorders, *Orthopaedic Surgery*, New York, Lippincott, Williams & Wilkins, 2001
4. Andersdon B. *Stretching, Revised Edition.* Shelter Publications, (pg 27-8, 47, 63-9, 95), 2000
5. Moore KL, Dailley AF. *Clinically Oriented Anatomy*, 4th ed. Baltimore, Lippincott, Williams, & Wilkins, 1999

6. Willis B, Burkhardt E, Walker J, Johnson M, and Spears T. "Preferential VMO Activation Achieved as a Treatment for Knee Disorders," *Int'l Jour Sport Med,* In Press, August 2002
7. Cutler JM: *Lateral ligamentous injuries of the ankle.* In Hamilton WS, editor. *Lateral* Ligamentous Injuries of the Ankle, New York Springer-Verlag, 1984
8. Prentice WE. *Rehabilitation Techniques in Sports Medicine*, 2nd Ed. Mosby, 1994
9. Rutheford OM. Muscular coordination and strength training. Implications for injury rehabilitation. *Sports Med.* 5:196-203,1988
10. Windsor RE, Dreyer SJ, Lester JP. Overuse injuries of the leg, ankle, and foot. *Phys Med Rehabil Clin North Am.* 5:207-213; 1994

11. Basmajian JV. Motor Learning and Control: A Working Hypothesis. *Arch Phys Med Rehab.* 59: 38-41, 1977
12. Cerny K. Vastus Medialis Oblique/Vastus Lateralis Muscle Activity Ratios for Selected Exercises in Persons With and Without Patellofemoral Pain Syndrome. *Phys Ther.* 75(8):672-83, 1996
13. LaDuke S. Untreated Pain: Could it land you in court? *Nursing 2002*, 23:9, pg 18, 2002
14. Micheli LJ. *The Sports Medicine Bible.* New York, Harper Collins, 1995

15. Levy AM, Fuerst ML. *Sports Injury Handbook.* New York, John Wiley and Sons, 1993

16. Moffat M. *The American Physical therapy Association: Book of Body Maintenance and Repair.* New York, Round Stone press, 1999

17. Adams P, Mylander M. *Gesundheit.* Rochester Vermont, Healing Arts Press, 1993

18. Rucker KS. *Chronic Pain Evaluation: A Valid, Standardized Assessment Instrument,* Boston: Butterworth-Heinemann, 2000

19. Maggie C. *Rehabilitation for traumatic brain injury: Physical therapy in context.* New York, Churchill Livingston, 1984

20. Mager RF. *Goal Analysis.* Belmont California, Lake Publishers, 1984

21. Adrian MJ, Cooper JM. *Biomechanics of Human Movement, 2nd Ed.* Madison Wisconsin, Brown & Benchmark, 1995

22. McArdle WD, Katch FI, Katch VL. *Exercise Physiology: energy, nutrition, and human performance,* 4th Ed. Baltimore, Maryland, Williams & Wilkins, 1996

23. MacKinnon LT. Current challenges and future expectations in exercise immunology: back to the future, *Med Sci Sports Exerc.,* 26:191, 1994

24. Guyton AC, Hall JE. *Medical Physiology, 10th Ed.* Philadelphia Pennsylvania, 2000

25. Drinkwater BL, et al. American College of Sports Medicine Position Stand on Osteoporosis and Exercise. *Med Sci Sports Exerc,* Vol 27:4, pg I-vii, 1995

26. Ayalon J, Simkin A, Leichter I, Raifmann S. Dynamic bone loading exercises for postmenopausal women: Effect on the density of the distal radius. *Arch Phys Med Rehabil.* 68:280-283, 1987

27. Hagberg JM, et al. Physical Activity, Physical Fitness, and Hypertension. *Med Sci Sports Exerc,* Vol 25:10 pg i-x, 1993

28. Kiyonga A, Arakawa K, Tanaka H, Shindo M. Blood pressure and hormonal responses to aerobic exercise. *Hypertension,* Vol 7, 125-131, 1985

29. Carpenter CL, Ross RK, Paganini-Hill A, Bernstein L. Breast Cancer and Exercise. *Br Jour Cancer,* 80(11): 1852-8, Aug; 1999

30. Luoto R, Latikka P, Pukkala E, Hakulinen T, Vihko V. Exercise decreases breast cancer risk. *Eur Jour Cancer* 36(6): 685-6, Apr 2000

31. Surgeon General. *Physical Activity and Health.* US Dept Health and Human Services, 1996
32. Rainey DL, Murray TD. *Foundations of Personal Fitness.* West Publishing Co., 1997
33. Williams ME. *The American Geriatrics Society's Complete Guide to Aging and Health.* Harmony Books, 1995
34. Baechle TR, Earle RW. (Editors) *Essentials of Strength Training and Conditioning.* National Strength and Conditioning Association. Human Kinetics 2000
35. National Institute of Health, National Cancer Institute, *SEER report,* 2000

36. Townsend M, Kladder V, Ayele H, Mulligan T. Systematic review of clinical trials examining the effects of religion on health., *South Med J.* 2002 Dec;95(12):1429-34.
37. Holy Bible, *New Living Translation,* Matthew 19:26

TERMS

1) <u>Abduction</u> – to draw away from the center of the body. Lifting one's arms away from the body is "abduction."

2) <u>Adduction</u> - to draw a limb towards the center of the body. Returning the arms to the side of the body is "adduction."

3) <u>Chronic</u> – persisting over a long period of time. An illness that has continued on the same level for over a year is "chronic."

4) <u>Closed-chained</u> – describes an exercise motion where the extremity is in full contact with a fixed surface. When doing a squat exercise, the foot is closed-chained because it is in fixed contact to the ground.

5) <u>Concentric motion</u> – this is the shortening of a muscle as the muscle fiber slides in contraction. When an arm is outstretched, and the biceps are flexed, the motion that brings the fist close to the shoulder is "concentric."

6) <u>Contract(ion)</u> – is the act of muscle filaments sliding past one another to shorten the total muscle length, but the filaments do not shorten. Contraction is like the sliding of a car's shock absorber. The two cylinders slide past one another to shorten the entire shock.

7) <u>Contusion</u> – is an impact injury where there is bleeding in the tissue beneath the skin.

8) <u>Coronal Axis or plane</u> – this is the plane or axis that runs from shoulder to shoulder.

9) <u>Dorsi flexion</u> – This is the ankle movement that lifts the foot and toes (as when letting up on the gas pedal, while driving a car).

10) <u>Eccentric motion</u> – this is a lengthening of a muscle (the opposite of concentric motion) and it occurs as the muscle fibers slide apart. After a biceps muscle contraction (elbow flexion),

the following extension movement of the arm with the muscle fibers sliding apart is "eccentric motion" for the biceps.

11) Isometric contractions – are contractions of muscle without movement of the limb. When one simultaneously flexes the biceps muscles and the triceps muscle, the arm stays stationary and is in "isometric contraction."

12) Open-chained – is an exercise activity where the limb is not in fixed contact with a surface. When one sits in a chair and straightens the leg with no resistance, it is an "open-chained" extension of the knee.

13) Orthotic – Is a device placed in a shoe or modified to be a fixed part of a shoe, and these devices are for correcting or changing alignment within the shoe, or for cushion, or to add length to a shorter leg. The goal of each orthotic is to give a person a smoother, healthier gait (walking pattern).

14) Plantar flexion – Is the ankle movement that points the foot and toes downward (like when accelerating the gas pedal in a car).

15) Plyometric – Refers to movement sequence that begins by eccentric (lengthening) of muscle, which is rapidly followed, by a concentric (shortening) contraction. Energy stored during the eccentric phase is rapidly recovered by the subsequent concentric phase. When a high jumper runs towards the bar, the final action is to jump to a squat, which lengthens the quadriceps muscles, then the quadriceps concentric contraction is more powerful.

16) Proactive – is the process of acting in preparation for a disorder or to use a preventative action to avoid a disorder or symptom.

17) Prone – Is the body position when the stomach is in contact with the ground or surface. Lying face down is prone.

18) Sprain - is an injurious stretch or tear in a ligament..

19) <u>Strain</u> - is an injurious stretch or tear in one's tendon.

20) <u>Subluxation</u> is the abnormal movement of a bone or joint, particularly in the lateral direction as with kneecap (patellar) subluxation.

21) <u>Supine</u> – is the body position of lying on one's back.

List of tables and figures

TABLES

FIGURES

List of Pictures

Complete Recovery and Rehab Success

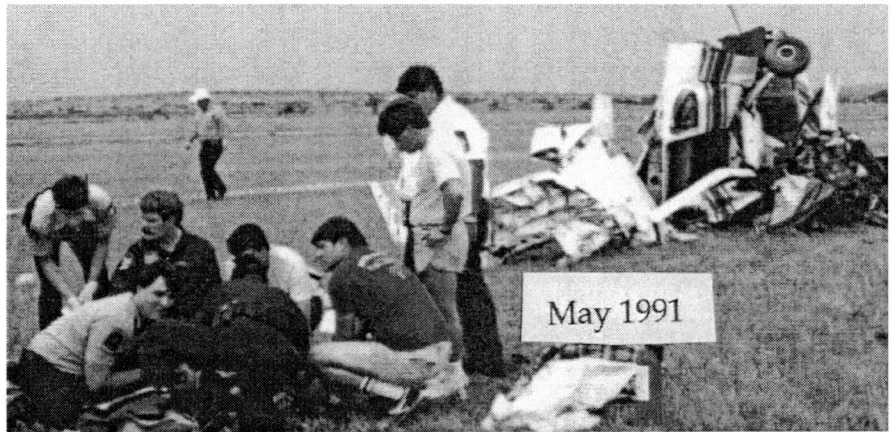

"Unsurvivable plane crash" (FAA comment 1991)

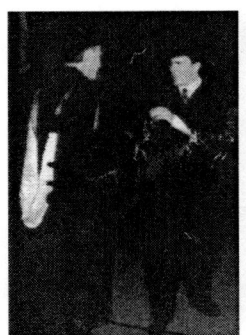

B.A. 1993

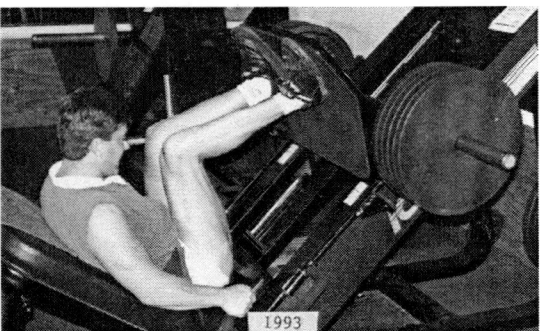

San Marcos Athletic Club, 1993

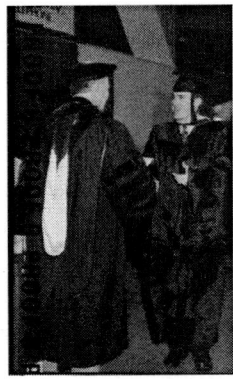

M.Ed. 1997

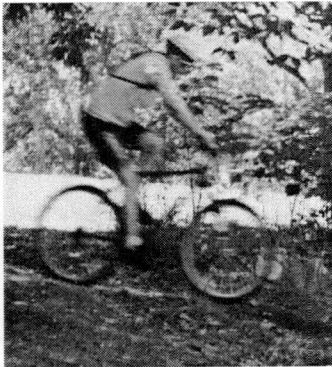

7th place MB race 1998

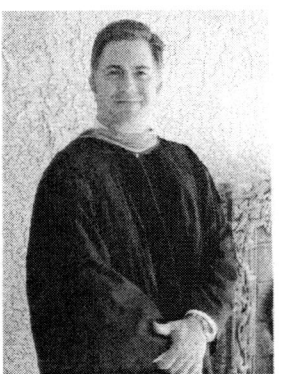

Ph.D. 2003

Thank you, God!

ISBN 1412005221-1